ALLERGIC
TO PETS?

Also by Shirlee Kalstone

Published by Bantam Books

HOW TO HOUSEBREAK YOUR DOG IN 7 DAYS

ALLERGIC TO PETS?

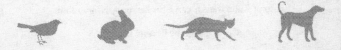

Shirlee Kalstone

Forewords by

Dr. Robyn Levy and Dr. Jeff Werber

BANTAM BOOKS

ALLERGIC TO PETS?
A Bantam Book / February 2006

Published by
Bantam Dell
A Division of Random House, Inc.
New York, New York

Library of Congress Cataloging-in-Publication Data

Kalstone, Shirlee.
Allergic to pets? : the breakthrough guide to living with the animals you love /
Shirlee Kalstone
p.   cm.
ISBN-13: 978-0-553-38367-4
ISBN-10: 0-553-38367-1
1. Allergy.   2. Pets—Health aspects.   I. Title.
RC585.K35 2006
616.97—dc22   2005053167

Printed in the United States of America
Published simultaneously in Canada

www.bantamdell.com

OPM   10 9 8 7 6 5 4 3 2 1

CONTENTS

ACKNOWLEDGMENTS

I wish to thank my husband, Larry Kalstone, and my agent, Joan Raines, for encouraging me to write about this complex subject, which affects the lives of so many pet owners. I hope the information herein helps readers to better understand what causes their allergies to pets, and how to manage them as effectively as possible.

I would also like to thank Shannon Jamieson Vazquez for pulling all the information together and making me look good. I couldn't have asked for a better editor.

Thanks as well to John Fry.

I am especially grateful to Dr. Robyn Levy and Dr. Jeff Werber, who took time away from their busy practices to read the manuscript and provide guidance, as well as to contribute the Forewords.

FOREWORD

Dr. Robin Levy
Board-Certified Allergist

I hung a postcard above my bed in college that read, "A dog is the only true love that money can buy," signed by Will Judy. I did not know who Mr. Judy was then, only that he knew whose love my money had bought. I've long since lost the postcard, but I never forgot the quote. The message has come back to me time and again over the past quarter of a century, as I've shared my life with the special dogs (and a cat) who have brought me more love, devotion, and smiles than I've ever paid for.

Any pet owner could easily substitute their favorite animal/pet/breed/lap dweller for "dog" in his quote and see the simple truth behind those words. We humans love our pets and they love us back unconditionally. This devotion is clearly demonstrated by the reported record numbers of pet ownership in America, and according to the U.S. Census Bureau, we spent more on our pets last year than on hardware, jewelry, and candy! Forty percent of us display a picture of our pets in our home (guilty), and 16 percent keep a photo of them in our wallet (also guilty).

When my mother and I were summoned to my pediatrician's office to discuss the results sent to him from the allergist who'd tested me the week prior, I remember him saying to my mother, "Dorothy, you'll have to get rid of the dog." She replied, "Doctor, we'll get rid of the child first." We kept our Dachshund (my best friend) and I got allergy shots for five years. And they worked: I had a relatively healthy carefree childhood, filled with lots of "dog and me" memories. I never guessed I would grow up to become an allergist, giving people the news daily that it is their beloved furry friend that is giving them or their child the fits of sneezing/itching/wheezing they so hoped was just from pollen. I have spent the last seventeen years gleaning all that I could from the little available medical literature on this subject, as well as from the veterinary world and often from my own allergic adult life experiences with pets (yes, the allergies came back), and from the feedback of countless pet-cohabiting patients.

I have learned that most allergic people don't have to give up their pets to gain significant symptom control. Also simple, inexpensive lifestyle changes at home can yield surprising results in helping to minimize pet-related allergy symptoms. And the changes and compromises patients make in their daily life, described so thoroughly and clearly in this book, can also bring about the added benefit of improved control with prescribed medications, as well as the need for fewer medications and less medically related expenditures, which we all want. It can be a win-win situation for the doctor, the patient, their family, and the pets.

There are certainly cases in which an individual may suffer from potentially dangerous allergic reactions to pets, such as severe swelling or difficulty breathing as in the case of some exquisitely sensitive allergic asthmatics. No one would argue that the danger to these individuals outweighs the need to have a furry or feathered animal in the home. Fortunately this scenario represents but a small minority of allergic sufferers, and even these individuals may be treated to tolerate occasional pet exposure outside of the home so that they can lead productive, predictable, and flexible lives.

For most allergy sufferers, newer medications afford acceptable symptom control. Allergy injections are effective in up to 90 percent of patients in helping to control or even eliminate symptoms. The latest generation of allergy medications currently in clinical use or in development have the potential to block allergic responses before they ever begin, rendering the recipient virtually "nonallergic"!

But the best measure against suffering from allergies to pets is minimizing exposure, which doesn't necessarily mean avoiding furry or feathered pets in the home altogether. Tolerable symptom control can often be achieved with minor alterations in the home environment. My own symptoms decreased dramatically just by buying my two Bassets their own warm, snuggly beds that are kept downstairs on hardwood floors, and keeping them out of the up-stairs bedrooms nearly all of the time. An even bigger change came about when I made the decision to get my pets out of my bed during my residency training. Each change came with some disappointed, guilt-inducing stares from my furry roommates, but over a short pe-riod of time, all adjusted (even me) and life (and rashes) got better.

I learned a great deal from reading this book that I can imme-diately apply to my patients' care as well as to my own pet-filled home. There is something for every type of pet owner in this book. It would be hard to imagine that any reader could not find at least one, if not many, practical and easy steps to enlist right away to make living with Fido (or Brittney, Lola, or Zeke) a healthier and thus happier experience. Read on, and enjoy learning how to live healthier with the "best love money can buy."

—Robyn J. Levy, M.D.

Robyn J. Levy, M.D., heads the Family Allergy & Asthma Center in Atlanta, Geor-gia. She is a board-certified allergist who specializes in the treatment of adult and pediatric allergy, asthma, and immunologic disorders. For more informa-tion about Dr. Levy and her work, please visit www.familyallergycenter.com.

FOREWORD

Dr. Jeff Werber, D.V.M.

When I finished reading this book, I thought ruefully, "Where was Shirlee Kalstone when I was a kid?" I sure could have used her expertise.

Growing up, all I ever wanted to be was a veterinarian. My folks said that ever since I was about five years of age, that's all I talked about. As a kid, we always had dogs but never cats. I inherited many things from my dad—some good and some not so great—but one of the worst things a kid could inherit from a parent, especially a kid who dreamed of becoming a veterinarian, was animal allergies. I tested positive for a number of foods, a plethora of pollens, and worst of all, cats, dogs, horses, sheep, goats, and cows! Would I ever consider changing my lifelong dream? Not a chance!

I never went through any phase of my life when I didn't have a dog. Cats, on the other hand, used to drive me nuts. Boy, do I remember the runny nose, scratchy red eyes, and the stuffed-up sinuses. And those crumpled telltale tissues. Everywhere. I was miserable and I was not pleasant to be around.

During graduate school, I began working as a technician at a local veterinary hospital, and fell head over heels for a little stray black cat with these magnificent green eyes. He was brought in by a hospital client who found him injured and unable to walk on his front right leg. We treated his wounds and got him back on his feet, and except for a mild residual limp, he was doing great. I became so attached to this little guy, whom I affectionately named Gimpy, that I decided to ignore my cat allergies and bring him home. Crazy or not, it was the best thing I ever did! I'm not sure whether having Gimpy around day in and day out provided me with a low-dose allergen that helped build up my immune system or if my allergies improved as I became a young adult, but suffice it to say that now I have no allergic sensitivities to cats! This is a very good thing considering I now have four cats to go along with my three dogs.

I can really empathize with those who have a tough time being around pets but refuse to give them up because they, too, suffer from animal allergies. Having practiced veterinary medicine for over twenty years, I have known countless pet lovers who suffered because of allergies yet still maintained their amazing relationships with their pets—those who have developed such a strong, meaningful bond with their four-legged or winged friends that they would not consider even for a moment giving up their loving companions. It has always amazed me that physicians or family members could even conceive of this possibility, much less recommend it in the first place. Pets are our kids, and we just have to deal with them and make room in our lives for them.

Well, for all you allergy sufferers—those who are currently braving the allergic reactions their beloved pets trigger or those who desperately want to experience the wonder of having them around—help is finally here! *Allergic to Pets?* is the most comprehensive single source of information for those of us who suffer from animal allergies. This book is packed with easy-to-understand explanations of what allergies are, how they affect us and our bodies, and more importantly, clear and comprehensive solutions to help us deal with and manage them. Whether you are sensitive to a tiny gerbil or dwarf hamster, a Lovebird or a Parrot, a dog or cat, or even a horse or goat, Mrs.

Kalstone offers clear and simple recommendations to help you cope with your allergies so you can enjoy being around your pet(s) even more.

Having worked so diligently over the years to enhance and celebrate the bond we share with our animal friends, I applaud Mrs. Kalstone for this fantastic book and consider it a must read for any animal lover who suffers from animal allergies.

—Jeff Werber, D.V.M.

Dr. Jeff Werber heads the Century Veterinary Group in Los Angeles, California, and is a nationally recognized expert on pets and their needs. Dr. Jeff, as he is affectionately known, practices outreach and education to promote and strengthen the bond between pets and their people. For more about Dr. Jeff and his work, please visit www.drjeff.com.

PET ALLERGY QUIZ

TRUE OR FALSE

The sensitivities that we know today as allergies were first recognized thousands of years ago by prominent Greek physicians of the ancient world such as Hippocrates and Galen. By the mid 1500s, Italian physician Pietro Mattioli recorded symptoms of a patient suffering from "cat fever," in what may be the first specific reference to pet allergy. He noted that the patient suffered agitation, sweating, and pallor in the presence of the cat, and reacted the same way even when the cat was concealed from him.

Scientific understanding of our immune system and what causes an allergic reaction is still rather recent, so it's not surprising that myths about pet allergies abound. Some are true; others are totally incorrect and frequently influence our attitudes and knowledge about dealing with sensitivities to pets. How many of these common beliefs about pet allergies can you identify correctly as true or false?

1. A pet's hair or fur causes allergies.
2. Short-haired dogs and cats may trigger fewer allergies than long-haired ones.
3. Kittens and puppies cause fewer allergy problems than adult pets.
4. You can be allergic to some breeds of dogs and cats and not to others.

PET ALLERGY QUIZ (cont'd)

5. You can become desensitized to your pet.

6. Dogs that shed excessively cause more problems for allergy sufferers.

7. Poodles, Bichons Frises, Maltese, and certain other purebreds are good choices because they shed little or no hair.

8. Cornish Rex, Devon Rex, and Sphynx cats are hypoallergenic because they don't shed hair.

9. Black cats trigger more allergies than other colors.

10. Some bird species can trigger more allergy symptoms than others.

11. Rabbits do not cause allergies because they are very clean animals.

12. Rodents and other small furry pets are recommended for allergy sufferers.

13. You can't ride horses if you are allergic.

14. Pets that live outdoors cause fewer allergy problems.

15. Restricting a pet to one or two rooms of your house will contain their allergens.

16. You can be more allergic to your pet in the spring and fall.

17. You can be allergic to clothing and furnishings made from animal fur or feathers.

18. People who are allergic to their pets must find new homes for their animals.

Answers

1. *False.* Allergic sensitization to pets is caused by dander, sebaceous skin gland secretions, saliva, and urine—*not* by hair or fur.

2. *True.* Although all dogs and cats—hairless, short-haired, long-haired, wirehaired, curly-haired, and even hairless—can trigger an allergic response, the shorter hair shafts of short-haired breeds usually carry less dander.

3. *True.* Baby animals have much less dead skin to shed and consequently little dander. They usually do not produce allergens in sufficient quantities to cause major sensitivities. However, from birth up to six weeks, while baby animals are nursing, they may temporarily be coated with more allergens due to their mother's licking and cleaning, and from the excessive amounts of urine in their whelping box.

4. *True.* Your tolerance level or sensitivity will not necessarily be the same to all breeds of dogs or cats. There can be significant variations even within a specific individual breed. For example, researchers at the Mayo Clinic found that some cats shed one hundred times more allergens than others of the same breed.

5. *True.* Many individuals can live comfortably with their own pets, probably due to natural desensitization related to years of exposure to their pets, but experience symptoms outside of the home.

Answers (cont'd)

6. *True.* All dogs shed, but double-coated breeds, like Akitas, Collies, German Shepherds, Samoyeds, and Shetland Sheepdogs, seem to cause more sensitivities than others. They have two kinds of hair: a thick outer coat and a softer undercoat. They can shed excessive amounts of hair, contaminated with allergens, throughout the home, especially during peak shedding seasons in late spring and early fall. There are also both single- and double-coated cat breeds.

7. *True.* No dog—purebred or mixed-breed—is truly hypoallergenic. However, Poodles, Bichons Frises, Maltese, Kerry Blue, Bedlington, and Soft-Coated Wheaten Terriers, Portuguese Water Dogs, and other breeds with soft, silky, or curly single coats, seem to be less allergenic. They have no undercoat, consequently they shed very little. Also, as many of these breeds require regular professional bathing and hair trimming, it can be easier for owners to keep them clean.

8. *False.* Even though Rex cats shed little hair and the hairless Sphynx cats shed no hair, they both still have dander, allergen deposits from their saliva, sebaceous gland secretions, and urine on their hair and skin, and in their litter boxes.

9. *True.* According to a report published in the December 2000 issue of *The Journal of the American Medical*

Answers (cont'd)

Association, cats with dark coats may provoke more allergic reactions than those with lighter-colored coats. Researchers found the odds for a reaction were six times higher with a dark cat.

10. *True.* Cockatiels, Cockatoos, African Grays, and Pigeons (known as "powder down" birds) can produce large quantities of white powdery dust on a daily basis. The powder becomes airborne every time a bird preens (runs its feathers through its beak), shakes its body, or ruffles its feathers, and can trigger allergic reactions.

11. *False.* While it's true that rabbits are very clean animals and make wonderful pets, they can cause allergic reactions because like cats, they constantly groom themselves with their tongues and coat their fur with saliva (a major pet allergen).

12. *False.* The spreading of allergens may be less of a problem with small furry animals that live in cages, but even they can trigger allergic responses.

13. *False.* Allergic individuals can ride horses, especially if someone else does the tacking up and the allergic individual mounts the horse outside of the barn. Horses themselves may not be the only source of allergens; sensitive individuals are often more allergic to mold spores and pollens in barns.

14. *True.* Taking a pet out of the home does help to reduce

Answers (cont'd)

the indoor allergen load, but it doesn't get rid of it entirely. The best alternative is to learn how to "allergy-proof" your pets and your house.

15. *False.* Isolating a pet to one or two rooms in the home does not fully contain their allergens, which can still be carried into other rooms on the owner's shoes and clothing, circulate naturally through the air, or spread via air conditioners, heating ducts, and fans throughout the house. However, keeping pets out of certain rooms, such as the bedroom, can significantly decrease the number of allergens that accumulate.

16. *True.* In most parts of the country, tree and grass pollens (in the spring and summer) and ragweed or other weed pollens (in the fall) are triggers of hay fever or seasonal allergic rhinitis. Individuals sensitive to both pets and pollens may find their pet-allergy symptoms are worse during pollen season because of double exposure to both types of allergens. Additionally, pets can carry pollen indoors on their coats, further exposing their owners to it.

17. *True.* Allergy sufferers can be sensitive to the animal fur and wool or feathers in clothing, fabrics, sweaters, glove linings, toys, cushions, blankets, and rugs. Items made of rabbit fur can be particularly irritating because the fur is too delicate to remove all traces of dander and

Answers (cont'd)

dried saliva. Feather- and down-stuffed pillows, comforters, and duvets also trigger allergic reactions.

18. *False.* According to an interview published in *Allergy & Asthma Health*, Robert A. Wood, M.D., director of the Pediatric Allergy Clinic, Johns Hopkins University School of Medicine, said, "There are no convincing studies demonstrating the direct clinical benefits of removing an animal from the home. No research has focused on whether finding a new home for a pet will eliminate the pet-related asthma or allergy symptoms." While symptoms may not go away, they can be very manageable. Most people with pet allergies can live with their pets if they take certain precautions that will minimize allergens on the pets themselves and in their homes.

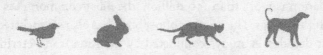

INTRODUCTION

Allergic to Pets? is about allergies to animals, specifically common household pets such as cats, dogs, birds, rabbits, gerbils, guinea pigs, hamsters, chinchillas, ferrets, rats, and mice, as well as horses. Allergy sufferers, and those who want to help relieve the suffering of loved ones, will learn about the following:

- Which pets cause allergies and why
- The allergic symptoms pets cause
- Reducing or eliminating pet allergies in the home and workplace
- Treating pet-related allergic skin conditions
- Minimizing allergens on hairy, furry, and feathered pets and their environments
- Allergen-proofing your home against animal, dust mite, mold, pollen, and cockroach allergens
- What professionals are doing to alleviate your symptoms

Pets have become an integral part of our daily lives and their populations are increasing throughout the world. In the United

States alone, pet ownership is at an all-time high: the total pet population is more than 150 million, the most common pets being cats and dogs. The number of pet birds has also skyrocketed in recent decades. A study[1] conducted by the American Veterinary Medical Association (regarded as the most extensive demographic study of pet bird ownership to date) estimates the current U.S. pet bird population at between 35 and 40 million. According to the Pet Industry Joint Advisory Council, in 1990 there were only 11.6 million pet birds—an increase of 245 percent! Unfortunately, sensitivity to cats, dogs, small furry pets, and birds is one of the allergies most frequently seen by physicians.

Statistics show that more than 50 million Americans suffer from allergic diseases, and a significant proportion of these people are also allergic to pets. Asthma sufferers are especially vulnerable: almost 30 percent are allergic to animals. It's almost impossible to escape exposure to animal allergens, for so many of us share our homes and even our beds with our pets. *A recent study found that even those who do not have pets in their own houses can have significant levels of animal allergens in their homes.*

The study[2] reported that inspections of homes in seventy-five locations across the country found allergens from cats and dogs in *every* home, even though these pets were present in fewer than half. "The implication of this for clinicians," the authors wrote, "is that they can be assured that *all* of their allergy and asthma patients have some home exposure to dog and cat allergens."

Many allergists routinely advise allergic patients to find new

1. *Journal of the American Veterinary Medical Association,* April 1998.

2. Arbes, Samuel J. et al. "Dog Allergen (Can f 1) and Cat Allergen (Fel d 1) in U.S. Homes: Results from the National Survey of Lead and Allergens in Housing." *Journal of Allergy and Clinical Immunology,* July 2004.

homes for their pets. More than 75 percent of owners disregard this advice, however, because it can mean a death sentence for a beloved animal, a decision that is impossible to contemplate. The Humane Society of the United States reports that in a study of hundreds of pet-allergic adults who were advised by their physicians to give them up, only one in five did. What's more, a large percentage of them obtained another pet after a previous one had died.

For allergy sufferers who do own pets, the human/companion animal bond is so strong that the thought of having to give up a pet because of allergies is almost impossible to contemplate. Intense emotional issues surface, especially when several children are involved and only one is allergic to a pet. It can be an even bigger issue between spouses or significant others.

Today, there is encouraging news for allergic pet owners. If you are one of the 75 percent of pet-allergy sufferers who prefer not to part with a beloved companion, this book will provide some effective alternatives. *But this book is not just for those who refuse to give up a pet, it's also for those who don't currently have pets and want to own one.* Although there is no cure for allergies, researchers have made dramatic advances in the understanding and management of airborne animal allergies in recent years. Allergic pet owners now have new environmental products as well as new approaches and treatment therapies to choose from. *Forgoing pet ownership or giving up a pet should be the last step an allergic person must take, not the first.* The trend has moved toward coexistence—establishing a plan that enables a person to keep his or her pet while taking certain practical steps to decrease the total levels of indoor allergens—and that is the purpose of this book.

ONE

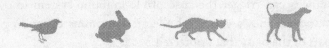

UNDERSTANDING ALLERGY
AND ASTHMA

According to the World Health Organization, allergies are the most widespread chronic condition in the world. There is no question that allergies are a major problem in this country. They are so prevalent that they affect almost every household. A great number of Americans either have allergies or know someone who does. In the United States alone, it is estimated that the number of people who suffer from allergies in one form or another may be as high as 50 percent,[1] costing them billions of dollars annually. And some doctors say these figures may be low estimates.

WHAT IS AN ALLERGY?

An allergy is a hypersensitivity or abnormal reaction to something that is ordinarily harmless to most people. Allergic reactions are caused by malfunctions of the immune system, the complex defense system that protects our bodies against invasion by bacteria, viruses, parasites, and other foreign substances or organisms that

---

1. American Academy of Allergy Asthma & Immunology. *The Allergy Report: Science-Based Findings on the Diagnosis and Treatment of Allergic Disorders, 1996–2001.*

threaten our health. A multitude of common, otherwise harmless substances can trigger the susceptible immune system to over-react and produce a variety of allergic symptoms depending on the part of the body that is affected.

Allergies can be inherited; if your parents or grandparents have a history of allergic sensitivities, you may develop allergy symptoms. If one parent has allergies, a child has a 20–40 percent chance of developing sensitivities; if both parents are allergic, a 40–60 percent chance. However, even though allergies can run in families, you can inherit just the *tendency* to be allergic, but not necessarily the same sensitivities that bother your parents. Allergies can also be influenced by a host of factors or conditions, such as geographical location, the time of the year, the climate and humidity, the pets you keep, the furnishings of your home or apartment, your housekeeping habits, what you eat or drink, the products you use, the drugs and medications you take, exercise, indoor and outdoor contaminants, and even your job.

Some allergies occur only at certain times of the year, while others are present all the time. Seasonal allergies coincide with the seasons when trees, grasses, and weeds begin to pollinate. The duration of the season depends on geographic location. Perennial, or year-round, allergies are usually caused by something you come into contact with every day of your life, including animal allergens, mold, and the droppings of dust mites and cockroaches. Since it is possible to be allergic to more than one allergen, many people suffer from both seasonal and perennial allergies.

WHEN DO ALLERGIES BEGIN?

Allergies usually appear before twenty years of age, and there is a tendency for them to start during early childhood. Young boys are more likely to suffer from allergies than young girls, but the pattern reverses itself in adulthood to affect women more than men. Allergies may change, they may come and go with no regularity, symptoms may wax or wane in intensity, or shift from one part of the body to another as a person progresses through different life stages, but the tendency to be allergic seldom goes away. Many individuals improve as years go on, but some do not.

THE IMMUNE SYSTEM

In her book *What's in the Air?*, Dr. Gillian Shepherd, clinical associate professor of medicine at Weill Medical College of Cornell University, has a most appropriate description for the human immune system. She calls it our body's "homeland defense system" and likens it to a giant network, similar to a road map showing many different routes, one of which leads to allergies.

Every minute of every day, a myriad of foreign invaders enter our bodies with no detrimental effects. Any foreign substance that causes the immune system to react is called an allergen (doctors also call these "antigens"). Allergens can be taken into our bodies in several different ways: via airborne substances we inhale; by food or drugs we ingest; by vaccines, medicines, and insect stings injected into our bodies; and through substances that come into contact with our skin.

Normally, when an allergen enters the body, the immune system springs into action and produces specifically programmed antibodies known as *immunoglobulins* to attack and destroy it. There are five different groups of immunoglobulins: IgA, IgD, IgE, IgG, and IgM. Each plays a different role that contributes to the functioning of the immune system. Immunoglobulin E, or IgE, is the antibody responsible for allergic reactions.

Along with IgE, three other types of body cells play a prime role in allergic reactions: *mast cells*, found in the tissues throughout the body (primarily in the mucous membranes of the respiratory and gastrointestinal tracts) and in the skin; *basophils*, a type of white cell (or leukocyte) found in the blood; and *eosinophils*, other special white blood cells.

THE BASICS OF AN ALLERGIC ATTACK

In an allergic person, the immune system learns to respond to one or more innocent foreign substances as if it or they were dangerous to the body. In the case of pets, for instance, the immune system perceives their dander, sebaceous gland, and salivary and urinary extracts as threats. Pet allergens are usually considered airborne allergens (though rashes caused by pet licking and contact dermatitis from pet dander are examples of non-airborne allergic reactions). Along with other inhaled substances such as pollens, mold spores, and the droppings of dust mites and cockroaches, they enter the body via the nose, throat, and lungs. Breathing them in can affect your entire respiratory tract. "For allergens to become capable of being inhaled, they have to be tiny— 1 to 5 microns," Dr. Shepherd says. "This means they are a millionth of a meter, or many times smaller than the dot at the end of this sentence."

The first step in the development of an allergic reaction is exposure to an allergen. Suppose, for instance, you have the potential to be allergic to cats. The protein cats produce that causes allergies in humans is called Fel d 1. Studies indicate that the sebaceous glands at the hair roots and the salivary glands are the most potent cat allergen sites. If you are a person destined to be sensitized to cats, when the tiny Fel d 1 protein comes in contact with your nose, lungs, eyes, or skin, your immune system reacts by producing specific IgE antibodies to this foreign substance.

Your initial exposure to the Fel d 1 cat allergen causes the IgE antibodies to bind in great number on the mast cells and basophils—many thousands may collect on a single cell—but you probably won't experience any symptoms. An allergen does not provoke a reaction the first time you encounter it. The immune system is simply gearing up to defend itself against future invasions by that same allergen. At this point, however, you are *sensitized* to cats.

Sensitization, or the process that leads to development of symptoms in persons intolerant to a particular allergen, requires exposure over a period of time—anywhere from hours, days, months, or years—to develop. Consequently, the second time your body encounters cat allergen (or maybe the tenth time, or the fiftieth time, or even the hundredth time) a sequence of biochemical reactions will occur culminating in the classic symptoms associated with airborne allergies.

When that occurs, and the Fel d 1 comes into contact with the IgE antibody that is produced to react against it, the mast cells and basophils attack the intruder and release a flood of destructive chemicals (the most important being histamine) into the surrounding tissues and bloodstream to trigger inflammation, either locally or systemically.

The union of an allergen and the IgE that takes place on the surface of the two cells is explosive. Several authors, in fact, have likened what happens to an explosion, comparing mast cells and basophils to grenades or land mines, and the IgE antibodies that bind to them to detonators. Depending on the tissue in which the "explosion" occurs, the allergic response differs. If the reaction to Fel d 1 occurs in the nose and throat, the responses can cause immediate swelling, itchiness, sneezing, a runny discharge, nasal congestion, an itchy or scratchy sore throat, and more. A similar reaction occurs in the lining of the eyes causing tearing, intense itching, and swelling. In the lungs, the muscles surrounding the air passages contract to make breathing more difficult, possibly starting the symptoms of asthma. If the reaction occurred from touching the cat, local swelling of the skin, itchiness, hives, or rashes may result.

This is not the end of the scenario, however. A few hours after the initial attack, in what is called the "late-phase reaction," eosinophils and additional basophils accumulate at the allergy site and release a host of inflammatory chemicals that contribute to both the severity of symptoms and the persistence of the attack.

THE CUMULATIVE OR "RAIN BARREL" EFFECT

Allergies are cumulative. In other words, they build up, and people can have varying sensitivities to different allergens. Every allergic person's immune system has a tolerance level above which symptoms will develop. This is often referred to as the "rain barrel" effect. Basically, when an allergic person's rain barrel is empty or partially filled, there are no allergic symptoms. However, when a combination of allergens, infection, and stress pile up, the rain barrel can fill up and overflow.

Someone who is allergic to a pet, for instance, may have no noticeable symptoms when the total exposure is below his or her tolerance level (the amount of substance or substances needed to provoke a reaction). That person may also have varying degrees of sensitivities to other substances found in and around his environment, such as dust, mold spores, pollens, soaps, cosmetics, and the like.

If a surplus of these allergens collect in the environment to exceed the allergy threshold, his or her rain barrel will overflow and symptoms will pop up. This being the case, while it may be impossible for you to entirely escape the effects of a pet in the house, taking proper precautions to lower environment triggers that are causing problems can significantly improve your tolerance of the pet or pets you live with.

ASTHMA

Asthma is an inflammatory disease of the lungs that causes airflow limitation and breathing difficulties. It is a serious lung disease that can be very disabling. Asthma may occur at any age, although it is more common in childhood. According to the American Lung Association, asthma is now an epidemic in the United States. In its "Trends in Asthma, Morbidity and Mortality," published in May 2005, the association reports that approximately 25 million Americans have asthma. The disease is responsible for 1.9 million emergency room visits, 12.7 million physician office visits, and about 13 million missed school days per year. As with allergies, genetics may play a role. A person is more likely to develop asthma if he or she has an asthmatic parent. The most common symptoms are wheezing when the sufferer is inhaling (although not all asthmatics wheeze), shortness of breath, and tightness in the chest.

Allergy can trigger asthma, although not all asthmatics are allergic and not all allergic people have asthma. In an attack, the bronchial tubes (the small branches in the lungs) become irritated. Cells release a cascade of histamine, leukotrienes, and other chemicals, causing the bronchial tubes to tighten and swell from the inside. At the same time, the muscles that encircle the outside of the bronchial tubes tighten and may twitch or feel ticklish (in medical terms this is called a *bronchospasm*), causing the airways to narrow. Mucus and fluids quickly accumulate in the lungs, narrowing the airways even further. This produces the tightness, wheezing, and coughing that are associated with asthma. Breathing more vigorously in an effort to maintain an adequate air supply and coughing up phlegm to relieve congestion can make your chest feel even tighter and make breathing *more* difficult.

When asthma is triggered by allergy, some of the allergens that are the culprits are the small dander, saliva, and urine particles of animals, bird-feather dust, house dust mites, pollens, and molds. Asthma can also be induced by a host of other causes such as exercise, emotions, cigarette smoke, air pollution, cold weather, foods, strong odors, as well as bacterial and viral respiratory tract infections.

IN CONCLUSION

Now you know a little about allergies in general. If you are looking for additional medical information, the bookstore and library shelves are stocked with books written by allergists and clinical researchers, filled with up-to-the-minute advice about managing allergies and asthma. Some are listed in the Resource Guide.

The rest of this book will zero in on sensitivities to pets: which pets trigger allergies; the allergic symptoms they cause; how to care for dogs, cats, birds, rabbits, and rodents and reduce your exposure to their allergens; plus how to allergen-proof your house to substantially decrease the number of dust mite, mold, pollen, cockroach, and other allergens in the environment. While it's impossible to rid your pet or your home entirely of animal allergens, you can *significantly* reduce their levels. Dr. William Berger writes in his book, *Allergy & Asthma Relief*, "No matter what the severity or cause of your condition, researchers have developed outstanding medications to end attacks and prevent new ones from occurring. Just as important, there are many, many things in your power to improve your situation."

TWO

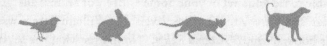

PET-RELATED ALLERGIC
SKIN PROBLEMS

Contact with any hairy, furry, or feathered animal can trigger allergic skin reactions in sensitive individuals. Skin conditions associated with pet allergens include hives (urticaria), angioedema (very large, swollen hives), atopic dermatitis (eczema), and contact dermatitis. Allergic pet owners can develop any of these by simply touching, fondling, hugging, or kissing their pets, and especially from being licked by their pets. In addition, close contact with dogs and cats that are infested with fleas can cause a skin rash called *papular urticaria*, which is an allergic reaction to the protein in flea saliva. In this case, you are not only allergic to your pet, but also to the fleas that live within the pet's coat. Here's a brief explanation of these conditions, how the skin reacts from contact with pets, and how doctors treat the symptoms.

HIVES AND ANGIOEDEMA

Hives are itchy, red, swollen bumps or welts on the skin that can appear soon after direct contact with a pet. The medical term for them is *urticaria*. They are always itchy and can also burn or sting. According to the Cleveland Clinic, hives vary in size (from a pencil eraser to a dinner plate) and can appear anywhere on the body after contact with a pet. They may look like mosquito bites, and can last for hours or up to three or four days before fading.

Angioedema is tissue swelling similar to hives, only it occurs in the deeper layers of the skin (around the eyes, lips, and hands), not on the surface. Unlike hives, angioedema is not itchy but can be associated with a painful or burning sensation and usually lasts longer than hives, although the swelling generally abates within 24 hours. Angioedema often appears with hives, but the two conditions can occur independently.

ATOPIC DERMATITIS OR ECZEMA

Allergy to pets can trigger *atopic dermatitis* or eczema in some people. It is characterized by red, dry, and itchy patches on the skin. Chronic scratching can thicken the shallow folds of the skin, giving them a leathery texture. The skin generally appears dry but some areas may be red and oozing.

ALLERGIC CONTACT DERMATITIS

When certain substances come into contact with the skin, they can cause an inflammation resulting in a broad range of reactions, including a fine rash, scaling, blisters, and burning sensations of the skin. Skin inflammation can be caused by an allergic reaction that involves the immune system while other causes are nonallergic irritants, such as cleansers or bleach. According to the American Academy of Allergy Asthma & Immunology, the hallmark of allergic contact dermatitis is that it occurs almost exclusively where the offending agents—allergens from the family pet, for instance— come into contact with the skin, like on the face after you hug your dog or cat, or on your hand or arm from saliva after being licked by your pet. Pets that go outdoors can carry poison ivy, oak, and sumac resins back indoors and that becomes another source of exposure for you.

TREATMENT

Basic treatment for all these skin ailments involves relieving symptoms and preventing further damage to the skin:

- Apply cool wet compresses directly to itchy skin.
- Avoid hot water. Take cool or lukewarm baths. Add a natural colloidal oatmeal, such as Aveeno, to the water.
- Use gentle soap, such as Basis Sensitive Skin Soap, or a soap-free cleanser like Cetaphil noncomedogenic skin cleanser.
- Blot, do not rub, your skin dry with a soft, clean terry towel.
- Lubricate your skin with hydrocortisone cream, moisturizing creams or lotions (Eucerin, Curél, Lubriderm, Keri, or other products recommended by your doctor) several times during the day, especially after bathing or showering, to prevent dryness. Avoid lotions that contain alcohol; they dry the skin.
- For hives and angioedema, over-the-counter antihistamines (such as Benadryl, Tavist, Chlor-Trimeton, or Claritin [Alavert] if drowsiness is a problem) can help to control itching. See a primary care physician for additional treatment if the rash is severe or does not respond to over-the-counter medications.

- For atopic dermatitis, your doctor can recommend over-the-counter topical preparations or can prescribe corticosteroids and oral medications to prevent scratching, depending on your condition. Antibiotics are prescribed if scratching has caused a secondary infection.

- For allergic contact dermatitis, your doctor may recommend over-the-counter topical creams or prescribe corticosteroids to stop the itching on small areas of the skin, and antihistamines or oral corticosteroids when larger skin areas are affected.

To prevent rashes and other previously described symptoms from recurring, it's best to avoid close contact with offending substances. Much as they may enjoy doing it, allergic children and adults should avoid hugging, kissing, and other close contact with their pets.

PAPULAR URTICARIA

In allergic individuals, intensely itchy, little red lesions from flea bites may pop up on the arms and legs and other uncovered areas, and occasionally across the stomach or shoulders. The lesions mature into firm reddish-brown bumps that are made worse by scratching. When fleas bite humans (as well as dogs and cats) they deposit saliva under the skin which causes the hypersensitivity.

Children—especially toddlers—tend to be more susceptible to these lesions because they usually come into closer contact with household pets when they cuddle them or roughhouse with them on the floor.

For proper diagnosis, you must first determine the presence of fleas. An easy way to do this is to wear white kneesocks and walk on your carpets or other suspected flea-infested areas for five minutes. If fleas are present, they will jump on the socks and will be easy to spot. Treatment varies depending on severity but may include topical steroid or antibiotic creams and antihistamines for severe itching. To keep from being bitten again, you must properly treat the pet to eliminate adult fleas, and also treat the environment to prevent fleas in preadult stages from developing. See chapter 5, "Minimizing Cat and Dog Allergens," for more information.

Whenever you notice an unusual rash, contact your allergist or dermatologist for assistance in treating and managing the condition.

THREE

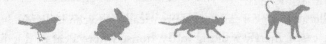

ALLERGIES TO ANIMALS

The primary focus of this book is allergic reactions to pets that live indoors (as well as horses) and secondarily, to the other indoor airborne allergens in our homes. As you read in the previous chapter, coming into contact with your pet can cause hives or a skin rash when you touch or otherwise handle the animal. More common, though, are sensitivities to pets from airborne allergens. Microscopic flakes of dried secretions from the animal's skin, saliva, and urine circulate through the air and, when you inhale them, your immune system shifts into overdrive to protect you. As a result, you sneeze and get a stuffy or runny nose, and suffer from other symptoms of allergic rhinitis.

Rhinitis is the most common allergy; millions of Americans suffer from it. Allergic rhinitis takes two different forms: seasonal and perennial. Seasonal allergic rhinitis is caused by sensitivity to pollens, trees, grasses, weeds, and airborne mold spores. Symptoms generally surface in spring, summer, or early autumn, depending on where you live. Perennial allergic rhinitis, as its name implies, is a year-round problem caused by sensitivities to a range of indoor allergens including dust mites, molds, cockroaches, and, most importantly for readers of this book, allergens from pets with hair, fur, or feathers. People can have both seasonal and perennial allergies.

Allergies to pets can vary dramatically between individuals. In some cases, merely walking into a house where a cat or dog lives may be enough to produce an allergic reaction within minutes. In other cases, an allergy can develop over time and exposure, and may not occur until a pet has been in your home for years. And occasionally, an allergic person develops a tolerance to symptoms and is able to live harmoniously with a pet, but why a specific individual becomes desensitized is not clear. An abstract published in 2003[1] reports that "increasing evidence shows that exposure to cats, dogs, and other animals can induce a form of immunologic tolerance without causing allergic disease."

THE ANIMALS THAT CAUSE ALLERGIES

Any warm-blooded animal with hair, fur, or feathers can cause allergies in humans at home or at work: cats, dogs, horses, rabbits, ferrets, gerbils, guinea pigs, hamsters, chinchillas, mice, rats, monkeys, goats, sheep, cattle, pigs and other farm animals, donkeys, mules, zebras, all species of large cats, and all kinds of birds, including chickens, turkeys, ducks, and geese. Cats, by far, cause the most allergic reactions, followed by dogs, rabbits, and horses. Let's focus for a moment on cats and dogs, the most popular housepets in the United States.

All cats and dogs—purebred, mixed-breed, short-haired, long-haired, wire-haired, curly-haired, and even hairless—are potentially allergenic. However, choosing the right cat, and espe-

1. Erwin, E.A., Woodfolk, J.A., Custis, N., Platts-Mills, T.A., *Animal Danders*. Immunology and Allergy Clinics of North America, August 2003.

cially the right dog, may make a big difference in successfully managing your child's, spouse's, significant other's, or your own allergies. What is important is not so much the length or amount of hair, but the quantity of hair that is or is not shed. All cats and dogs (except hairless breeds) shed, but those that shed excessively seem to trigger more sensitivities, due to the excessive amount of allergens the dead hair may carry. And when pets have an illness or skin condition that leads to excessive shedding, more dander is temporarily produced. Most people think short-hairs don't shed much around the house but, in fact, they shed a great deal and can spread as many allergens into the environment as pets with medium or long hair. Others may have more problems with double-coated pets (a longer outer coat with soft undercoat), especially dogs that shed profusely. Pets with soft, curly, or silky hair (with no undercoats) seem to cause fewer allergy problems.

While some animals may produce more or less allergens than others, *there are no "hypoallergenic" cats or dogs*. We know that some dogs and cats produce far more allergens than others but the differences are not specific to any particular breed. In fact, studies have found that the differences in allergen production within a single breed can be as great (or even greater) than the differences between multiple breeds. Studies also show that allergen production is controlled by hormones: males produce more allergens than females, and when males are castrated, the amount of allergens produced decreases within a month. Still, according to Dr. Robert A. Wood, of Johns Hopkins University, "It is not possible to predict with any accuracy which animals are likely to be more or less allergenic based on a particular breed, size, hair length, or propensity to shed."

Animals that *do not* disperse allergens into the environment and are nonirritating are those with no hair, no fur, and no feathers: fish, snakes, turtles, lizards, frogs, toads, and so forth. These are the only "safe" pets for allergy sufferers. But be aware of the mold that can accumulate on damp fish tank lids.

IDENTIFYING THE MAJOR ANIMAL ALLERGENS

There are several sources of pet-related allergens, all accomplishing the same end: being inhaled into your lungs and triggering allergic or asthmatic reactions. They are:

- Secretions from the sebaceous glands of the skin, located at the base of the hair follicles. These are oily lubricants that keep the skin supple; they are deposited on the hairs inside the follicles and brought up to the surface of the skin along the hair shaft.

- Saliva spread on hair or fur when an animal licks or cleans itself.

- Urinary secretions that are frequently deposited on the hair, especially on long-coated animals.

All these are liquid proteins that are microscopically small, and light enough to remain airborne almost indefinitely. Equally important is an animal's dander—dead particles that shed regularly from the skin and are similar, but much smaller in size, to skin cells that exfoliate from your own body and scalp. Combine all these particles and you virtually load your home with pet allergens.

Pet hair itself is *not* an allergen; it merely serves as a carrier. The sebaceous gland, salivary, and urinary allergens dry on the hair and subsequently flake off into the environment, along with dander, to become airborne for extended periods of time. They also enter the environment on contaminated hair that pets shed, particularly when they are being stroked or groomed, when they shake, vigorously wag their tails, jump on furniture, chase balls, or play indoors, and when they rub against objects.

Pet allergens, particularly those of cats, are infinitesimally tiny in size—literally invisible to the human eye. They are extremely light in weight; they circulate on air currents throughout the house, floating in the air for hours before eventually settling into carpeting, soft furnishings, rough-textured fabrics and wallcoverings, heating ducts and air conditioners, and anything else they come into contact with. Once they do settle, walking on or vacuuming the carpets, sweeping floors, sitting on the furniture, fluffing up cushions or the pet's bedding, raising or lowering the blinds, and opening or closing drapes or curtains causes tremendous amounts of allergens to billow into the air once again. Even when allergens that have settled are not disturbed, there is an ongoing low level of exposure.

Cat and dog allergens are also easily transported on clothing and shoes, thereby spreading to public places such as schools, hospitals, office buildings, shopping malls, hotels, cinemas, buses, and trains.

The longer a pet lives in a home, the more its allergens will have permeated the entire house to cause symptoms. And when cats or dogs have lived in homes for a long time, their allergens can be deeply embedded in carpets and furnishings even *after* many cleanings. Cats and dogs often share their owners' beds and this, too, increases the level of exposure to their allergens; numerous studies have shown there to be huge accumulations of them in bedding and mattresses.

Although isolating a pet to one or two rooms in the home may lower the level of exposure somewhat, doing so only contains their allergens to a limited degree; currents throughout your home, such as forced-air heating, air-conditioning, and fans can spread them throughout the premises. Keeping a pet outdoors or finding it a new home isn't a foolproof solution either. Researchers at Johns Hopkins University have found that it is not uncommon for animal allergens to remain in a home for surprisingly prolonged periods of time after an animal has been removed.

SOURCES OF PET ALLERGENS

The following are believed to be important sources of pet allergens:

Animal	Allergen Sources
Cats	Sebaceous gland secretions/saliva/dander/urine
Dogs	Dander/sebaceous gland secretions/saliva/urine
Birds	Feather dander or "dust"/droppings
Rabbits	Saliva/dander/urine
Ferrets	Urine/dander
Gerbils	Dander/urine*
Guinea pigs	Urine/saliva/dander
Hamsters	Urine/dander
Chinchillas	Urine/dander
Mice and rats	Urine
Horses	Dander/urine

* Although rodent urine is allergenic, gerbils are desert animals that excrete small amounts. Nevertheless, their urine may be an allergen source.

DOG AND CAT ALLERGENS PRESENT IN 100 PERCENT OF U.S. HOMES

Actually, complete pet allergen avoidance may not be possible at all. A study published in the July 2004 *Journal of Allergy and Clinical Immunology* found that even when allergy sufferers don't own a dog or a cat, but live in communities with a high prevalence of pet ownerships, their pet allergen exposures at home will likely be above allergic sensitization thresholds.

The study found that although a dog or cat had lived in only 49.1 percent of the homes, *their allergens were detected in 100 percent (dog) and 99.9 percent (cat) of homes.* The highest allergen concentrations were found on living room sofas. In homes with pets, the higher level on sofas could reflect where pets prefer to spend time, as well as the persistence of allergens on upholstered sofas which are difficult to clean. In any home, however, it likely reflects the site most likely to come in contact with clothing worn outside the home. Even in homes where a dog or cat has never been present, their allergens had to have been passively transported inside.

THE ALLERGIC SYMPTOMS PETS CAUSE

Allergy symptoms generally develop along the path the allergens follow as they enter the body: animal allergens involving the respiratory tract may cause many different kinds of symptoms in people, depending on where the mast cells release histamine and other irritating cellular products. The severity of reaction to these allergens varies from one person to another, and they can also be intensified by simultaneous allergies to other airborne irritants in the environment. The most typical symptoms are:

- Red, watery, and/or itchy eyes
- Itching of the nose and throat
- Watery nasal discharge, sometimes alternating with nasal congestion
- Postnasal drip
- Sneezing (sometimes multiple times in rapid succession)
- Scratchy palate and throat
- Chronic sore throat
- Shortness of breath, difficulty breathing, or wheezing
- Itchy skin, hives, atopic or contact dermatitis produced by touching a pet or being licked by one

ALLERGIES TO CATS

Cats cause more allergy problems than other animals and sensitivities to them can be serious. Cat allergen is one of the most potent of all allergens. Some people cannot enter a house or apartment where a cat lives, or even has lived in the past, without rapidly developing symptoms.

The sebaceous skin glands, the salivary glands, and dander are the primary sources of the major cat allergen, a glycoprotein called Fel d 1 (or *Felis domesticus 1*) by clinicians. Fel d 1 is also found in their urine, blood, and tears, as well as in the female cat's milk. It is said that an average cat sheds 0.2 grams of hair and dander each day, causing high concentrations of Fel d 1 in the house.

Why Cats Cause More Problems Than Other Pets: Their Tiny Fel d 1 Allergens

Published studies show unequivocally that Fel d 1 is associated with small particles that remain airborne for long periods—hours to days—in contrast to larger particles of dust mite, cockroach, dog, pollen, and mold allergens that settle to the ground within minutes and only become airborne when disturbed. Fel d 1 is about ten times smaller in size than dust mite or pollen particles, ranging in size from 1 micron to about 15 microns, with a significant percentage being about 2.5 microns in diameter. What size is a micron? As an example of just how small one is, *the period at the end of this sentence is nearly 1,000 microns in diameter.*

To a cat-sensitive individual, this means that because Fel d 1 allergens are microscopic in size, they can easily float throughout the house, even without air disturbance. They are extremely "sticky" when they do settle and cling stubbornly to walls, furniture, carpets, and drapes. They affect the eyes quickly; they are instantly inhaled in significant quantities into the lungs to set up a chain of immune-system events that produce the symptoms described earlier in this chapter.

Some authors have claimed saliva to be the principal source of Fel d 1, but a study conducted in Marseille, France,[2] to determine the importance of saliva and sebaceous glands as sources of the Fel d 1 allergen, dramatically demonstrated that the cat's skin is the most abundant source. The study compared the Fel d 1 levels at the base and tip of the hair on (a) the belly where sebaceous

2. Mata, P., Charpin, D., et al. Department of Chest Disease and Allergy, Hôpital de Ste-Marguerite, Marseille, France. "Fel d 1 Allergen: Skin and or Saliva? Annals of Allergy," *October 1992.*

skin glands are sparse but licking is frequent; (b) the axillary area (armpits) where both sebaceous glands and licking are infrequent; and (c) the base of the tail where sebaceous skin glands are numerous and licking infrequent. If saliva was the principal source of allergens, then the belly should have produced the most Fel d 1. But the results showed that there was much more Fel d 1 at the base of the hair than the tips; in fact the base of the tail, which had the most sebaceous skin glands and the least amount of saliva, had twice as much Fel d 1 as the others.

It's not only domestic house cats that are potentially allergenic. All the members of the cat family, including lions, tigers, leopards, jaguars, panthers, pumas, and ocelots are known to affect veterinarians, zookeepers, circus performers, and others the same way.

Feline Self-Grooming: How Saliva Is Spread

Cats are notoriously fastidious. They groom themselves repeatedly by licking their fur with their tongues and occasionally removing bits of matted fur and debris trapped in the hair with their tiny front teeth. This methodical self-grooming is not just a matter of personal hygiene; it is a reflex behavior in normal, healthy cats. Unfortunately for cat-allergic individuals, they deposit large amounts of saliva on the hair with each lick of their tongues, which dries, sloughs off, and becomes airborne to trigger allergic symptoms.

The tendency to lick themselves begins around the second or third week of kittens' lives. As they mature, self-grooming becomes increasingly significant, and it is estimated that most adult cats spend 30–40 percent of their waking time cleaning and grooming themselves. Self-grooming achieves several purposes: removing loose hair, dust, and debris; cleaning the fur and skin; and stimulating the skin glands to spread natural oils throughout the coat to keep it waterproof. It also plays a role in temperature control. Like other animals that do not sweat through their skin, cats spread excessive amounts of saliva onto their fur and skin where it evaporates and cools them down in warm weather.

A cat's tongue is ideally suited for self-grooming, being covered with numerous hard, sandpapery barbs that slant backwards toward the throat. Cats have extremely flexible spines and can convolute themselves into all sorts of positions to reach nearly every part of their bodies with their tongues; for those parts they can't reach, like the head and the neck, they liberally lick a forepaw and use that to rub across the neck and over the face and ears. *They literally coat themselves with saliva.* Along with grooming themselves, cats occasionally use their tongues to groom humans. Licking their owners' skin is a comforting behavior linked with kittens that were separated too early from their mothers. Unfortunately, this behavior can cause a skin rash when the allergens in the saliva come into contact with an allergy sufferer's skin.

Rubbing

Dried Fel d 1 particles are also shed into the environment when cats rub themselves against objects. Rubbing is a form of feline scent-marking and communication. It's the cat's way of claiming territory by "marking" favorite individuals, other pets, and inanimate objects such as doorways, chairs, and furniture. In the process of rubbing against people, other pets, or objects with their chins and foreheads, cats transfer glandular secretions that humans can't smell but other cats can. These become an olfactory stimulus to other cats that might pass by, saying, for instance, "Stay away! This chair is *mine*."

HYPOALLERGENIC CATS?

Allerca, a Los Angeles-based biotechnology company, is attempting to produce "hypoallergenic" cats that are expected to be available sometime in the future, at a cost of $3,500 each. The British Shorthair was chosen as the first breed of hypoallergenic cat. The new felines will be the product of genetic engineering that, the company claims, will "silence" the gene that produces Fel d 1. According to Allerca's president, the cats will not be totally allergen-free, but the small amounts remaining are reportedly not enough to trigger reactions. Every kitten sold will be spayed and neutered to prevent breeding with naturally born animals. Allergy specialists are skeptical until more widespread exposure to these animals over longer periods of time can be examined.

ALLERGIES TO DOGS

Like cats, the major cause of allergic reactions to dogs is not the hair but the proteins that are secreted by the sebaceous skin glands, the saliva that is deposited onto the hair and skin when the dog licks itself, and dander. The major dog allergens are called Can f 1 and Can f 2 (or *Canis familiaris 1* and *2*). Urine is also a source of dog allergens, but dander and saliva are the major culprits. When these secretions dry on the hair, they flake off—like the tiny allergens cats shed—and float in the air throughout the house. In addition, according to the American College of Allergy, Asthma & Immunology, exposure to dogs that have been running in fields during pollen season and then come back into contact with their owners has been reported to cause acute symptoms of allergic eye inflammation, as well as hay fever due to secondary exposure from the pollen on their coats.

The possibility of breed-specific allergens has been studied for years and, while findings have demonstrated variations in quality and quantity of extracts derived from different dog breeds, *no single breed has been found more or less allergenic than others.*

Dogs and Dander

Animals constantly shed dander (dead skin cells) as their outer layer of skin (or epidermis) turns over or regenerates itself. The epidermis is made up of multiple thin layers which are constantly pushing upward from the deepest level of the epidermis to replace the cells above. This process is called *epidermal turnover time.* In a normal dog, this process takes about twenty-one to twenty-two days. As the new cells make their way to the surface, the dead ones flake off as dander. These tiny dead particles are usually contaminated with sebaceous gland secretions, saliva, or urine, which increases their allergenicity.

Variations in Epidermal Turnover in Dogs

In *Small Animal Dermatology,* Drs. Muller, Kirk, and Scott indicate that trimming the hair with clippers shortened the epidermal turnover to approximately every five days instead of the usual twenty-one. They also report that epidermal turnover has been shown to be even more rapid—three to four days—in dogs with seborrhea, a chronic skin disease characterized by excessive scale formation. Seborrhea takes primarily two forms: dry, known to affect Irish Setters, German Shepherds, Doberman Pinschers, and Dachshunds, and oily, which typically affects Cocker and Springer

Spaniels, West Highland White Terriers, Basset Hounds, and Chinese Shar-Peis. In the oily form, the skin and hair coat are greasy to the touch (a film often remains on one's hand after stroking the coat), excessively scaly, and have a strong odor. From an allergy standpoint, this means that seborrheic dogs with a rapid epidermal turnover produce much more dander than those with a normal fifteen- to twenty-one-day turnover. It is important to have a veterinarian diagnose these conditions and implement treatment to bring them under control. Cats, incidentally, only occasionally develop seborrhea, possibly because they remove dead skin scales during self-grooming.

ALLERGIES TO BIRDS

Birds are also growing in popularity as pets. The *Statistical Abstract of the United States* reports that nearly one in twenty pet-owning homes have birds. The most popular pet caged birds belong to two zoological orders, Psittaciformes and Passeriformes. Psittacine birds are members of the Parrot family and include Cockatoos, Cockatiels, Budgerigars/Parakeets, Lovebirds, African Grays, Amazons, Macaws, Lories, and Lorikeets. Passerines are the "perching" birds, the various Canaries, Finches, Sparrows, Mynas, and over half of the known living bird species, many recognized for their singing abilities.

All birds, especially "powder down" birds (primarily Cockatiels, Cockatoos, African Grays, and Pigeons) can produce allergic reactions in humans. The major bird allergen is derived from their feather dander or dust. The feathers themselves have little allergic potential. When birds preen themselves and flutter their wings, no matter how small they may be, they shake feather dust into the air and in and around their cages. Feathers that have molted and small feather particles that break off during playing or exercising also collect around bird cages. All these are very light; they become airborne easily and circulate throughout a house by way of air currents, air-conditioning, and heating ducts. Bird droppings, too, can be a source of bacteria, fungi, mold, and dust.

Bird Feathers

Every bird has several different kinds of large and small feathers. Each serves a specific purpose, including flight, insulation, waterproofing, and protection. Some of the different feather types include contour, semi-plume, filo-plume, down, and powder down.

Bird feathers are made from a hard protein called *keratin*—similar to the keratin your hair and nails are made from. Feathers, with the exception of powder downs, are not permanent on birds; they are shed and replaced by new ones on a regular basis through a process called *molting.* Molting is controlled by hormones and occurs one or more times a year, depending on the species. In pet birds, the frequency of molting can be affected by age, diet, humidity, temperature, seasonal changes, and stress, as well as dryness in centrally heated homes.

Once worn feathers have molted, or shed from their follicle in the skin, new feathers, coated with keratin, grow in the same follicle. As the feathers mature, the keratin breaks off into small pieces to produce feather dander or dust.

The Preening Gland

Most birds have a preening gland (also called the uropygial gland) located at the back of the base of the tail. The preening gland secretes an oily substance that birds spread throughout their feathers with their beaks. During preening, a bird gently rubs its beak against the gland and strokes along the barbs of each feather, starting at the quill (the part embedded in the follicle below the skin) and working up to the tip, spreading oil over the feathers to groom and arrange them. Birds can't reach their heads with their beaks, so they scratch oil onto their heads with their claws. Among other things, preening is important for waterproofing and keeping the skin and feathers supple. As preening makes the feathers a little sticky and causes them to become matted, to properly maintain their plumage, birds like to bathe regularly to wash off the excess oil. Bathing is another way loose feathers are shed.

Powder Down Birds

While all birds produce feather dust that can trigger allergies, some members of the psittacine family, on which the preening gland is small or absent altogether, produce *significant* amounts of powder on their feathers. These powder down birds—specifically Cockatoos, Cockatiels, African Grays, and Pigeons—*cause the most irritation to people with allergies, asthma, and other respiratory problems.*

Powder down feathers are small and downy with brush tips that help to insulate a bird. Unlike other feathers, powder downs grow constantly. Instead of being molted, the tips or barbs disintegrate into a fine, slightly waxy, white talcumlike powder, composed of keratin, which the bird spreads through its feathers. This action aids in lubricating and waterproofing the rest of the plumage. In the wild, the powder prevents rainwater from gaining access to the skin through the feathers.

Powder down birds are extremely dusty and produce much more feather dust than other birds. They may cause serious problems for people who are allergic to birds because they can produce enough powder to coat the floors, furniture, and most other surfaces of the room in which they are caged on an almost daily basis. If you stroke a powder down bird, you'll usually come away with a coating of fine white powder on your hand. Unfortunately, this dust is so minute that it quickly spreads and circulates throughout the house.

Extrinsic Allergic Alveolitis or Pigeon Lung Disease

People who live or work with caged birds or pigeons are susceptible to a respiratory condition known as extrinsic allergic alveolitis (EAA) and by the more popular name of pigeon or bird fancier's lung disease, caused by a reaction to inhaling fine dust from a birdcage or aviary. EAA takes three forms: acute, subacute, and chronic. The chronic form is the type most pet bird owners develop; the main symptoms are progressive difficulty in breathing during physical exertion, chronic dry cough, and decreased lung function. Exposure to low doses of bird allergens over long periods of time can cause chronic EAA.

There is no correlation between the severity of the illness and the number of birds a person keeps, and it has been reported that a single Budgerigar may cause the same degree of illness as four hundred in a home aviary in a hypersensitive individual. Canaries, Budgerigars, Finches, Lories, Lovebirds, Macaws, Mynas, Parakeets, pet Pigeons, and especially the powder down birds kept in homes have been documented to be the sources of allergens.

Untreated, EAA can cause permanent and serious lung damage which will remain long after the bird is gone. For mild cases, giving up all contact with birds or aviaries may be all the treatment that is necessary. More serious cases are generally treated with oral corticosteroids, often combined with other anti-inflammatory drugs. If you keep birds, seek immediate medical attention for any respiratory irregularities.

Even If You Don't Own a Bird

Allergies to birds can also occur without the presence of live birds in your home via the use of feathers in bedding and clothing. A study conducted in Finland demonstrated that true feather allergy is extremely rare and that most of the reactions seen in skin prick tests to feather extracts are principally caused by dust mite allergens present in the feathers.[3] Therefore, while allergy sufferers should avoid using feather pillows or down comforters, more importantly, they should invest in special mite-proof encasings and comforter covers to reduce exposure to dust mites.

ALLERGIES TO SMALL FURRY PETS

Rodents, rabbits, ferrets, and other small furry creatures have become increasingly popular as household pets of both children and adults. They are small, easy to care for, and inexpensive to feed, don't bark or squawk to annoy the neighbors and are often permitted in many apartment complexes where dogs and cats are prohibited. However, even though many of these pets are caged, their urine, dander, and saliva are still allergenic. The amount of allergens they create depends on their size, how many pets there are, how often their cages and bedding are disturbed, how often they are handled by family members and, in the case of rabbits and ferrets, whether they have the run of the house. Also, since mice, rabbits, and other small furry pets such as hamsters or gerbils often are kept as classroom pets, keep in mind that schools can be overloaded with pet allergens.

3. Kilpio, S., et al., Lappenrata, Finland. "Allergy to Feathers." *Allergy* 53, no. 2 (February 1998), pp. 159–64.

Studies indicate that urine from mice, rats, guinea pigs, hamsters, chinchillas, rabbits, and ferrets contains allergens that can trigger reactions. It appears that proteins present in the urine, particularly of males, are the primary cause of allergies in rodents. High levels of urine allergens in rodents have been well documented by veterinarians, laboratory workers, and research scientists. And mites living in rodent feces and in cage linings can aggravate sensitivities, especially when changing or cleaning the cages.

Additional allergens from dander and saliva have also been identified that, in the case of gerbils, guinea pigs, and rabbits, are significant. In fact, the allergens in rabbit saliva and dander are of major importance. Rabbits have become increasingly popular in recent years, as more people discover that they make superbly adaptable pets. Rabbits are intelligent, can be successfully trained to use a litter box, and are often allowed free run of the house. Like cats, rabbits groom themselves repeatedly by licking their fur, and each lick of their tongues during the self-grooming process deposits saliva on their fur which dries, eventually flakes off, and becomes a source of airborne allergens.

ALLERGIES TO HORSES

Horses are extremely allergenic animals, even though they do not live indoors. The most important sources of horse allergen come from their dander and urine. Horses also have a high sweat rate; this produces the characteristic strong "horsy" odor which greatly aggravates allergies. Sweating helps horses lose heat when their body temperature increases due to exercise. They sweat more when the weather is hot and less when it cools. Sensitivities to horses are very troublesome and not well understood, because practically everything associated with horses and their environment can lead to allergic reactions. For instance, horses eat hay and oats and graze on grasses, which are all potential allergy triggers. They spend much of their time confined in barns and stables, where mold spores may be growing in damp hay and pollens from ever-present grasses can trigger allergies. Horses also love to roll in dusty or muddy places, to rid themselves of

PETS MAY PROTECT CHILDREN FROM ALLERGIES

Here's some *good* news about pet allergies. Recent evidence indicates that persistent exposure to high levels of dog and cat allergens may have a protective effect against the development of an allergy among both boys and girls. Despite the age-old belief that exposure to cats and dogs in a home can be a leading cause of childhood allergies, a study published in the October 2003 *Journal of Allergy and Clinical Immunology* indicates that the opposite may be true. Dr. Thomas Platts-Mills, M.D., Ph.D., of the University of Virginia, and Swedish researchers studied children in northern Sweden, ages seven to eight years, for several years and found that, despite cats being the most common sources of allergens, keeping them in homes was *not* related to an increased risk for sensitization. The longer children kept cats and dogs when they were young, the lower the incidence of developing allergies to these animals compared to new pet owners and to those who had only been exposed briefly. In fact, among those who were allergic to cats, 80 percent had never had a cat at home.

dead hair and parasites, and vigorously shake out their thickly powdered coats, which can aggravate allergies. The tanning agents and lanolin waxes used on their bridles, harnesses, and saddles, as well as the wool in their saddle blankets, can also trigger allergic contact dermatitis. Additionally, once someone becomes sensitized to horses, they can also be bothered by horsehair found in old furniture, rug pads, and mattresses. Fortunately, using horsehair as stuffing material is not as popular as it once was.

The good news is that some patients who think they are allergic to horses are actually mold-allergic and do fine if someone else does tack work for them and they mount the horse once it is outside of the moldy barn.

FOUR

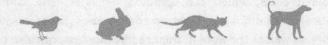

GENERAL SUGGESTIONS FOR REDUCING ALL PET ALLERGENS

While totally eliminating the substances that trigger symptoms may be ideal, sensitivities to animals and other airborne allergens can be relieved by "allergen-proofing" both your pets and your home.

The steps you take depend primarily on the severity of your allergies. To get effective relief, of course, people with serious allergies and asthma will need to take more definite measures than those with mild sensitivities. "Healthy coexistence of allergic owners and animals is possible, if the humans are prepared to go to a little extra trouble," says Dr. John Ohman, chief of Allergy Division, Department of Medicine, Tufts University–NEMC. Thanks to research from around the world, we now have a much better idea of the actions that can be taken and the products that are available to help alleviate allergies to pets and to airborne substances.

The first logical step to control your sensitivities is to minimize exposure to pet allergens and other airborne allergens that exceed your tolerance threshold, thereby making your "rain barrel" overflow, and triggering attacks. Preventing exposure is the first line of defense.

This chapter gives you some general suggestions on how to reduce exposure to all pet allergens. The chapters that follow zero in on specific animals: cats and dogs, birds, rabbits, rodents, ferrets, and horses. Chapter 12, "Allergen-Proofing Your Home," includes room-by-room steps for effective environmental control to make your home as allergen-free as possible.

One of the most important ways to control the dispersal of allergens into the atmosphere is via regular grooming and cleansing of pets, and keeping their bedding or cages fresh and clean. According to the Humane Society of the United States, simply brushing and cleansing a pet regularly can reduce the level of allergens on the hair by as much as 85 percent. Remember, it's not the pets themselves that trigger your sensitivities. It's the dander, the sebaceous and salivary glands, and urinary secretions that dry on their hair and contaminate their environments that provoke reactions.

When pets are neglected, and not brushed or cleaned at least once a week, microscopic particles of their allergens become airborne in large quantities. As mentioned in an earlier chapter, pet allergens, especially Fel d 1 from cats, are extremely light and buoyant, and float freely on air currents throughout a house, making it just about impossible for any room to be entirely "safe."

Proper fresh and clean housing is also of great importance, especially for birds and small animals that live in cages. A cage must not only meet the spatial needs of the pet, but must also be easy to clean. The longer urine, fecal matter, spoiled food, and dirt remain, the greater the chances the cage will become contaminated with allergens, become a breeding ground for disease, and a potential health danger to you and your pet.

GENERAL SUGGESTIONS FOR ALL PETS

Here are some general recommendations that can help to decrease your exposure to animal allergens. Specific advice concerning each of the animal species follows this section. Please read carefully before going on, as these pertain to *all* pets, and will not be tediously repeated in each individual chapter.

- You can avoid spreading allergens by scrubbing your hands and arms *immediately* after direct contact with your pet—handling, stroking, hugging, or kissing it, for instance. You may also want to wash if your pet deposits saliva on your skin; many people develop symptoms and rashes after being licked by a dog or cat.

- Brushing, combing, and cleansing the hair, fur, or feathers regularly (at least once a week) are important to remove dander and any loose dead hair or feathers contaminated with pet allergens.

- Bathe or cleanse your pet on a *weekly* basis to reduce the amount of dander. Bathing does reduce the amount of allergens, but the results are only temporary. A study[1] published in the 1997 *Journal of Allergy and Clinical Immunology* found that washing cats with soap and water did reduce allergens, but the reduction didn't last longer than a week.

1. Avner, D.B., Perzanowksi, M.S., Platts-Mills, T.A. "Evaluation of Different Techniques for Washing Cats." *Journal of Allergy and Clinical Immunology,* September 1997.

- To avoid the hassle of a bath, you might use a pet allergy relief solution (such as Allerpet, Dander-Off, or AllerFree) to simplify the weekly cleansing. The majority of cats will prefer this to the extremely distressing bath. These products are applied to pets, usually on a weekly basis, to help reduce allergic reactions in humans. Of the various pet allergy relief solutions on the market, Allerpet is the only one to be scientifically tested. It cleanses the skin and hair of dander, saliva, and urine allergens by controlling their dispersal into your environment, and by conditioning and moisturizing the skin and hair to reduce future accumulations. A study[2] conducted at Eindhoven University in the Netherlands, presented as an abstract at the 1995 American Academy of Allergy Asthma & Immunology (AAAAI) annual meeting, found that the treatment showed a decrease in removable Fel d 1 allergen in treated cats, as well as a decrease of nearly 50 percent in detectable Fel d 1 in settled dust.

- In addition to cleansing birds, rabbits, and small furry rodents of the allergens that trigger symptoms, their cages should be scrupulously cleaned at least once a week to discourage the buildup of dander, dried salivary and urinary secretions, molds, and bacteria. Allergens that dry and accumulate on bedding and cages become airborne when these reservoirs are

2. Koren, Wiet. "The Effect of Allerpet/C Treatment on Fel d 1 Concentrations in Settled Dust, Cat Fur and Air." *Journal of Allergy and Clinical Immunology*, February 1995.

disturbed. Have a nonallergic family member do these jobs. If possible, and the cage is not heavy, take it outside for cleaning, then let it dry in the sun.

- When you stroke or otherwise handle your pet, your clothing also collects allergens that the animal sheds. Choose something washable to wear when you brush or cleanse your pet, and if the pet sits in your lap, spread a towel across your legs to prevent loose hair and fur from clinging to your clothing or to furniture.

- Launder the towel that you spread over your lap and grooming clothes as soon as you finish, or at least put them in a separate basket or hamper. Don't spread the allergens throughout your home, especially into your bedroom.

- If possible, a nonallergic family member should do the grooming or cleansing, outdoors ideally, or in a well-ventilated area like a screened porch (so that all the dead hair and dander loosened by the brush or comb won't end up circulating throughout the house). If this is not feasible, then the allergic person should wear a protective mask (available from local medical supply houses or mail-order allergy supplies catalogs listed in the Resource Guide) while grooming or performing any clean-up duties, as well as when dusting, mopping, or vacuuming, tasks that can agitate settled allergens.

- Avoid contact with soiled litter boxes or rodent cages.

- Ask your veterinarian for recommendations for a balanced diet and skin supplements for your pet. The right diet or the addition of a skin supplement may help to minimize shedding and hair loss. Dry skin, accompanied by excessive flaking, is a common problem of cats and dogs that live in homes with forced-air heating or that are poorly ventilated.

- In addition to the various pet allergens, hair can also collect dust, pollen, mold, and other irritants which is another reason for cleansing. When dogs and cats go outdoors and walk through grassy or weed-strewn areas, the outdoor allergens their hair collects can be an irritant for pollen-sensitive children and adults *even if they are not allergic to the pets themselves.* It's a good idea to lightly moisten a washcloth with water or an allergy cleansing product and wipe over the pet's hair to remove as many allergens as possible, as soon as they come indoors.

- The type of clothing you wear can affect the transportation of pet dander. Researchers at the University of Sydney found that people who wore wool sweaters were exposed to more than ten times the amount of Fel d 1 than individuals wearing no upper body clothing. People who wore freshly washed T-shirts were exposed to the least amount of cat allergen. Clothes made of textured fabrics collect pet allergens easily; they should be laundered frequently.

- *Keep pets out of the bedroom!* Adults spend one-third of their day (and children up to half their day) in their bedrooms. Never allow dogs and cats to sleep on your bed, and do not keep the cages of small, furry pets or birds in the bedroom. According to the WebMD medical library, when pets are removed from bedrooms, the allergens in the air decline by 70 percent. Close the door during the day to discourage pets from napping on your bed. Experts say that when allergy sufferers breathe *pure* air for eight to ten hours each night, they can probably tolerate more exposure to allergenic substances during the day.

- Pet allergens (along with dust mites) collect in large quantities in pillows, blankets, and mattresses. Encase all bedding in protective coverings. See chapter 12, "Allergen-Proofing Your Home."

- Train dogs and cats to sleep in their own beds (with washable cushion or blanket), away from your bedroom. Wash their bedding regularly in hot water (check manufacturer's care suggestions) and tumble dry to eliminate pet allergens plus any pollens that come indoors on the pet's hair. Launder dog sweaters and clothing, as well as fabric collars, occasionally. Vacuum the pet's bed and the surrounding area often.

- Wash plastic, rubber, and nylon toys, as well as flying discs, with hot water and mild dish soap to remove saliva, a major allergen. Rinse well and dry with a clean cloth.

- Restrict your pet's presence in dens and living rooms with carpets and soft furnishings, as nothing traps animal dander like rugs and upholstery. "Having cat allergens building up in the carpet and furniture is like living with twenty cats," says Thomas Platts-Mills, M.D., head of the Asthma and Allergic Diseases Center at the University of Virginia. If your dog or cat has a favorite chair or couch that you don't want to declare as off-limits, cover it with a sheet, a throw, or plastic cover (wash the sheets/throws weekly). Better yet, if possible, confine pets to areas of the home without carpets or upholstered furniture.

- Check out the various pet hair pick-up rollers, magnets, and foam-latex dry-cleaning sponges that clean without water. They act like erasers, attracting embedded pet hair from clothing, upholstery, lamp shades, bedding, drapes, and carpets. Most rollers have easy-to-grip plastic handles with perforated tape sheets. You simply roll over the item to be cleaned, tear off and dispose of the sheet, and replace it with a new one. Other extra-wide tape rollers have handles that adjust up to 48 inches long to collect hair from drapes, stairways, floors, or anywhere you might need extra reach.

- HEPA (High-Efficiency Particulate Air) or ULPA (Ultra-Low Penetration Air) filters can be a big help in removing allergen particles, especially Fel d 1. HEPA filters purify 99.97 percent of all airborne particles larger than 0.3 microns in diameter. ULPA filters absorb and contain 99.999 percent of all airborne particles larger than 0.12 microns. Standing or tabletop units are available for use in individual rooms or filters can be adapted to your central HVAC system. Read more about air filters in chapter 12, "Allergen-Proofing Your Home."

- Wash walls and other surfaces regularly. This is significant if you own a cat because the cat allergen

Fel d 1 is sticky. Once it settles, Fel d 1 adheres to walls and other surfaces in enormous quantities.

- Proper ventilation and air circulation will also help to lower the concentration of pet allergens. Poor air distribution throughout the home is a major factor contributing to the buildup of indoor airborne allergens, pet odors, mildew, and the resulting health problems. EPA studies indicate that indoor air is often more polluted than outdoor air. To encourage natural ventilation, whenever the weather is suitable, unless the allergy sufferer is sensitive to outdoor allergens or the air is polluted, open several windows (screened, of course, to prevent pets from escaping) for a short time each day to draw fresh air inside.

FIVE

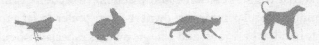

MINIMIZING CAT AND DOG ALLERGENS

Cats, by far, cause the most allergic reactions, followed closely by dogs. Although cats and dogs are considered almost essential to the American family experience, allergic responses can create intense conflicts, especially if only one family member is allergic and the others are not. You can decrease the amount of pet allergens in your home by simply paying better attention to your cat or dog: grooming regularly, cleaning its hair once a week via a bath or the use of an allergy cleansing solution, keeping it free of fleas, making sure that a dog is housebroken or a cat litter box trained, keeping it out of your bedroom, purifying the air with a HEPA[1] filter and keeping the dust mite population to a minimum.

GROOMING HELPS TO REMOVE ALLERGENS

All short-haired and long-haired cats and dogs need to be groomed regularly—not only to keep them looking beautiful, but

---

1. HEPA, or High-Efficiency Particulate Air filters are made of densely packed glass fibers that are pleated to increase their surface area and particle-trapping ability. They remove at least 99.97 percent of the particulate matter of 0.3 microns or larger from the air. See chapter 12, "Allergen-Proofing Your Home".

also, and more importantly to allergy sufferers, to minimize the allergens that trigger reactions. Many dog breeds require complex trimming at regular intervals; owners often prefer to let professionals handle these jobs, and allergic owners especially should.

Between appointments, or in the case of dogs and cats that are not regularly groomed by a professional, the following procedures for brushing, combing, and cleansing the hair will help decrease the pet allergen load in your home.

Brushing and Combing

Even if you are not allergic, brushing and combing is one of the most essential aspects of taking good care of your pet to keep the skin and hair clean and healthy. For allergy sufferers, brushing or combing *at least once a week* is even more important because it removes dander, foreign matter, dirt, and loose dead hairs that are contaminated with dried salivary, sebaceous gland, and urinary secretions, and keeps them from shedding into the air and spreading throughout your home.

Establish a regular brushing and combing routine as soon as possible. The sooner you start, the easier it is to get your pet accustomed to the process. There are many different kinds and textures of dog and cat hair, and each coat type has its specific requirements. You need the correct brush and comb; your pet supplies dealer or the breeder from whom you purchased your pet can recommend the right tools.

If you are allergic, try not to brush your pet yourself. Let a family member do the job (outdoors when possible). If you must do the grooming yourself, cover your nose and mouth with a mask. Before you begin, put a little water into a spray bottle and lightly moisten your pet's hair. Brushing dry hair increases the chances that dander and loose contaminated hair will fly all over the place.

The basic premise of "allergen-proofing" is to *brush all the way down to the skin*, not just the top of the coat, to loosen and remove dander and dead hair. This is easy to do on short-haired dogs and cats but requires more effort when the hair is longer. The best way to handle long hair is to brush small areas at a time. Use your fingers to separate the hair into small sections. Hold the unbrushed hair out of the way with your free hand, and brush each section from the skin outward with gentle sweeping motions. Once your dog or cat is completely brushed, comb through the coat to check that all loose dead hair is removed and there are no tangles. Remove the hair that collects in the brush and comb frequently and deposit it into a waste basket nearby. When the session is finished, wash the brush and comb. Change and launder your clothes.

Shedding

Brushing and combing pets regularly is a year-round essential for allergy sufferers. For dogs and cats that shed heavily, it helps to prevent an excessive amount of dead hair from piling up throughout your house. While no breeds are "hypoallergenic," people may have more problems with animals that shed profusely because of the excessive amount of loose hair—contaminated by dander, dried saliva, and urine—that falls off the pet and into your carpets, upholstered furniture, bedding, and clothing.

The shedding process is normally triggered by the lengthening and shortening of daylight patterns that signal the changing of seasons. When cats or dogs live in unheated natural conditions, they usually shed twice a year, in the spring and in the fall. Continuous indoor living disrupts the natural shedding cycle, however, and pets that are exposed to more artificial light than sunlight shed all year round, though the process does become more extensive in the spring.

When this happens, especially on Collies, German Shepherds, and other densely coated breeds, the undercoat loosens and starts coming out in chunks. Persians and other long-haired cats also shed profusely. You *must* help nature along by removing the loose dead hair, *especially in the spring,* before your household furnishings are covered with it! A washable grooming glove is an especially helpful item at this time. Various kinds, with flexible rubber tips or plastic nibs, help to grab and remove loose dead hair as you "massage" your dog or cat. Your pet will love the attention and probably won't even realize he's being groomed.

Hairballs in Cats

The shedding of hair can cause an additional and more serious problem in cats: hairballs. You learned in chapter 3 that cats are notoriously fastidious and groom themselves repeatedly by licking their fur. The surface of a cat's tongue is composed of rough, backward-slanting papillae which collect and hold the loose, dead hair during the licking process. Once this happens, the hair cannot be expelled, so the cat swallows it, and it ends up in the stomach, where it can accumulate and form into a mass called a "hairball."

Many cats have no problems with hairballs whatsoever; others are especially prone to them, such as long-haired cats and cats that groom excessively. If the hairball doesn't pass through the stomach, the cat will usually cough or gag in an attempt to bring it back up through the mouth. If the cat cannot regurgitate the hairball, however, a blockage can form in the stomach or small intestine which can become a serious problem. Treatments designed to break up hairballs include a cat food with a hairball control component, treats containing mineral oil, and petroleum-jelly-based lubricants and laxatives that you can put on your cat's paw to be licked off. Serious hairball problems should always be referred to a veterinarian. For cats that are prone to hairballs, frequent brushing helps to reduce the amount of hair that is ingested. The more loose hair you can remove by brushing your cat, the less hair he will swallow.

Bathing Cats and Dogs

Allergy sufferers can also reduce sensitivities by bathing their pets or by wiping the pet's coat with an allergy cleansing solution once a week. Properly performing either procedure on a regular basis will not harm your dog or cat.

Bathing once a week *temporarily* reduces the amount of allergens on a pet. The earlier in life a cat or a dog becomes used to a bath, the better the chances of having it accept the process without becoming panic-stricken. Most dogs learn to accept (and even enjoy) being shampooed. Cats, on the other hand, may only tolerate baths and giving one is not an experience for those who are faint of heart or short-tempered. If you've tried washing your cat unsuccessfully, wiping over the coat with a pet allergy solution can be an alternative to the dreaded bath.

Where to Bathe

Where you bathe—bathtub, laundry tub, sink, or shower stall—depends on your pet's size. Resign yourself to lots of spilled and splashed water at first. Pets often become frightened when they stand on slippery surfaces; a rubber mat or nonskid strips on the sink or tub bottom will secure footing and ease tension. Placing a folded terry cloth towel under a cat's feet is a good way to anchor them if you're dealing with a whirling dervish or escape artist.

If you need to protect yourself from your cat's claws, wrap a few strips of nonstick first aid or surgical tape snugly around the paws so that the toes cannot be spread or the claws extended. The tape usually falls off by the end of the bath; if it does not, simply pull it off in the direction the fur grows and it will not cause any harm.

Steps Before the Bath

Assemble all your supplies in advance: spray attachment or a plastic cup for wetting; hypoallergenic shampoo, crème rinse, or conditioner (for long-haired pets); and several large terry cloth towels. There are many fine hypoallergenic shampoos formulated for dogs and cats. Don't use a human shampoo—select one that is pH balanced for pets, as both dogs and cats have more alkaline skin and hair—and *don't* use dishwashing soap. If your pet has a special skin problem, you'll want a recommendation from your veterinarian.

Always brush and comb your pet's hair before the bath. Bathing matted hair only makes matters worse as shampoo residue, dead hair, dander, and other pet allergens get trapped in the tangles and are nearly impossible to rinse out. Don't forget to let your pet go outside or use the litter box before his bath.

Giving the Bath

For dogs: turn on the water and, as soon as it runs consistently warm, *not hot,* stand the pet in the tub.

For cats: it's best to fill a large plastic dishpan or the sink with about two inches of warm water, add a little shampoo, swirl it around with your finger and *then* put in the cat. Bathing most cats the first few times is a job for two people—one to hold and control, the other to wet, shampoo, and rinse. But if you must handle a fussy feline alone, face your cat *away* from you, so that if an escape is attempted, the cat will leap up and try to claw the air, not you. Grip the scruff of the neck firmly with one hand while you wet and shampoo with the other. Using a nylon harness and leash is also a good restraint.

When you begin bathing your dog or cat, wet the hair thoroughly all over except for the head and ears, either pressing the sprayer directly against the coat to propel the water down to the skin, or pouring the water over the coat with a plastic cup to remove as much dirt and loose dander as possible. It takes time to wet hair, especially for pets with thick, almost water-resistant coats. Cat hair, especially, tends to resist wetting; pouring sudsy, rather than plain, water over the cat helps to moisten its coat faster.

Bathing a pet is like bathing a baby. Speak lovingly and reassuringly as you wet the hair, praise your pet, and say its name often. Shampooing from back to front and washing the head last often helps to give more confidence. Nothing will spook a nervous animal more than wetting its face as soon as it goes into the tub.

Apply shampoo, using your fingertips or a sponge to work up lather, and wash the body, legs, and tail. On cats, pay particular attention to potentially greasy areas, such as on top of the tail and behind the ears. Wet and wash the head last. Use a washcloth to clean the face; take care not to get shampoo into the eyes. If your pet is very dirty or has long hair, rinse lightly and shampoo a second time to make sure the hair is extra clean.

Rinsing: The Key to a Clean Dog or Cat

Begin the final rinse at the forehead, then spray or pour water methodically down the neck, back, over the sides of the body, down the legs to the feet, and over the tail. Hold the spray nozzle or cup *close to the skin* and rinse thoroughly to remove all traces of shampoo and, *more important, all loose dander, Fel d 1, and urine residue.* Keep rinsing and rinsing until clear water rolls off the coat. Squeeze the excess water from the hair, blot any wet areas inside the ears with cotton, wrap the pet in a towel, and take it out of the tub.

Drying the Hair

Continue blotting the coat with dry towels to absorb excess moisture. Keep your pet in a warm area, away from drafts, until the hair is completely dry. Dogs and cats with long or thick coats can take a long time to dry naturally; you may want to use a hair dryer to speed the drying process. Wear a mask if you plan to blow-dry the hair. Launder all towels used to dry your pet as soon as possible.

Using an Allergy Cleansing Solution

Using an allergy cleansing lotion in place of a bath is also an effective (and much less aggravating) way to temporarily remove allergens from a dog's or cat's coat and skin, especially for pets that behave like wild animals during a regular bath. Allergy cleansing solutions are lotions that are applied to cats and dogs (and birds and small furry pets as well) to help reduce allergic reactions in humans.

The pet allergy solution can be applied with a damp washcloth once a week. If your pet is small, you can wipe it on while the animal sits in your lap. Just spread a large, clean terry towel over your lap for your pet to sit on. This will keep you dry and prevent hair (coated with allergens) from shedding onto your clothes.

Dampen a washcloth and lightly wipe your pet from the skin outward, first against the lay of the hair, then with it, until all areas are damp, *not dripping wet,* to remove loose dander and dried saliva and urine. Wipe several times over the areas your pet licks most often—around the genitals, for instance, where urine tends to collect and dry on the hair. No rinsing is required. Dry the hair thoroughly with a towel or hair dryer. Launder your grooming clothes and all towels used in the process.

FLEAS CAN MAKE YOUR ALLERGIES WORSE

Although all animals with hair and fur are susceptible to fleas, they are the most common external parasites of cats and dogs. Fleas, tiny wingless insects that possess powerful leaping abilities, are more than just irritating because they can cause allergies and disease in not only pets but also in people. Fleas are parasitic insects with piercing/sucking mouth parts that bite pets and feed on their blood. Their strong, springy legs make it easy for them to move freely from dog to dog, from cat to cat, from cat to dog, and even from pet to human!

Dogs and cats themselves can be allergic to the saliva that fleas deposit under their skin as they siphon blood. Pets can become so irritated that they scratch themselves raw, resulting in flea allergy dermatitis, a condition that requires veterinary treatment.

A study conducted at the University of South Florida found another important reason for allergy sufferers to pay close attention to fleas: flea debris, including eggs and body parts, can circulate in the air and cause allergic reactions in people. The study found that *the impact of flea debris may be as significant as that of pollen.* While collecting dust samples in the homes of allergy patients, a large number of them had fleas and, in some cases, they were actually leaping out of the dust samples during examination.

Looking for Fleas?

It's not easy to see fleas, but if you part your pet's hair to the skin and look closely, you can spot them scurrying through the hair if the pet is infested. Their favorite hangouts are the groin, under the front and back legs, on the head, and behind the ears. Even when you can't see them, you can tell if your pet has fleas by noticing little black specks about the size of pepper or poppy seeds in the coat—"flea dirt" or waste matter. If you rub these onto a damp paper towel, the smear will turn deep reddish brown because they contain blood digested from your pet.

You may also learn that your pet is infested with fleas by being bitten yourself. They tend to bite humans mostly on the arms and legs, but bites can occur anywhere, especially if an infested pet sleeps in its owner's bed (see "Papular Urticaria," pages 17–18). Unfortunately, if one pet in your household has fleas, chances are all other pets do too.

The Flea's Life Cycle

Fleas have a tremendous capacity for reproduction. Ten adult females can, theoretically, produce a quarter of a million offspring in one month and millions by the second month! Experts say that for each flea you spot on your dog or cat, hundreds more in pre-adult stages are hiding in your house, waiting to become adults and hop back onto your pet.

Treatment and Prevention

To successfully combat flea problems, *you must treat your pet, your pet's bedding, and your indoor environment immediately.* If the pet goes outdoors, you may also need to treat the lawn, patio, or other areas where the pet spends time. If you own more than one pet, you must treat all dogs and cats in your household.

Flea control products come in many forms, including collars, powders, sprays, foams, shampoos, dips, "spot-on," "sponge-on," and tablets. Before you purchase or use any of them, talk to your veterinarian, who is the best source for current flea control data.

Some of the new topical and systemic oral treatments that are available are safer to use, more effective, and environmentally friendlier than ever before. Topically applied solutions called "spot-ons," including Advantage, Frontline, and Revolution, come in plastic squeeze tubes, and are applied directly to the pet's skin between the shoulder blades, where they are absorbed into the skin and spread throughout the body. Spot-on products work by killing adult fleas on the pet before they have a chance to lay eggs, and are effective for up to a month or longer.

Systemic adulticides or insect growth regulators (IGRs), including Program and Sentinel, are administered orally on a monthly basis. These do not kill adult fleas, but work by killing emerging larvae.

Flea shampoos containing natural pyrethrins also are among the safest and most effective products to use. However, natural pyrethrins are derived from certain species of the chrysanthemum family. These are closely related to ragweed, public enemy number one for allergy sufferers. Discuss this matter with your veterinarian if you're allergic to ragweed.

Whatever you use, follow package directions precisely, especially for cats. *Cats are not small dogs.* They can be especially sensitive to medications and chemicals and quickly develop toxic reactions. Call your vet immediately if you notice an adverse reaction, or contact the ASPCA Animal Poison Control Center at 1-888-426-4435.

Treating Your Home

In addition to treating your dog or cat, wash your pet's bedding in hot sudsy water. Bedding that is heavily infested needs to be replaced. Thoroughly go over all carpets, upholstered furniture, floors, baseboards, cracks and crevices, and all your pet's favorite areas with a vacuum. Dispose of the vacuum bag as soon as you have finished, or else it will become an incubator for newly hatched fleas. If you can't throw away the bag, add a little flea powder or chopped up pieces of flea collar inside.

You should also steam-clean carpets and flooring to reach hidden eggs and immature forms, especially around baseboards or anywhere there might be corners or cracks. Washing pet bedding, vacuuming, and steam-cleaning can still leave live fleas and other chemical treatment may be necessary. Check with a licensed pest control company about choices, as they use a variety of insecticides and know which products work best indoors and outdoors in your area.

IS YOUR PET HOUSEBROKEN OR LITTER BOX TRAINED?

If you own a dog, *be sure it is completely housebroken.* If you own a cat, *it should always urinate in a litter box if it doesn't go outdoors.* Urine, as mentioned in an earlier chapter, is a trigger of symptoms for people who are allergic to pets. Along with allergens in pet urine, allergy sufferers can also overreact to strong urine odors, especially when secretions have dried on carpets or hard surfaces.

Dogs and cats that are not housebroken or litter box trained make the problem worse. The smell of old urine in a home is nauseating, and becomes even worse during humid or rainy weather.

When ignored, urine may seep through the carpeting into the padding and floor underneath. Male urine smells the strongest, but females can excrete pungent odors, too, and the older the pet, the stronger the odor. Cat urine is said to be the worst source of odors and stains.

The mention of pungent-smelling cat urine would not be complete without a word about urine spraying. Do not confuse normal urination, which occurs when cats squat and lower their hindquarters and urinate on horizontal surfaces (even outside of a litter box) with urine spraying. When cats spray urine, they stand erect, facing away from the object to be sprayed, hold up their tails, and forcefully eject a stream of urine on walls, furniture, and other vertical surfaces. Urine spraying is more common in males, especially those living in multicat households, and mainly concerns territorial boundaries.

When unneutered male cats reach maturity, at around seven or eight months, they become possessive about their territory and begin to spray urine to mark it. They spray on vertical surfaces at a level that other cats can easily smell to send a message that a certain territory is occupied—for instance, "Stay off this couch, it's my property." The pheromones and fatty ingredients in the urine, especially of males, leave an obnoxious odor that can be extremely sensitive to allergy sufferers. If you have a male cat, you may want to have him neutered. Ninety percent of male cats stop urine spraying within several weeks to months after being neutered. And when the procedure is performed before sexual maturity, most cats never begin to spray.

What Causes That Awful Smell

Ammonia, mercaptans, and other chemicals and gases emitted from urine (and feces) cause the odor. Once a pet urinates on a surface, the urine begins to decay: the urea breaks down into ammonia and, in a second stage, produces mercaptans and other gases that give rotten cabbage and skunk spray their obnoxious smells. You may clean and clean contaminated surfaces, but if you don't eliminate the smell, the odor of stale urine becomes stronger over time. Meanwhile, the aroma entices your dog or cat back to re-soil the same place again and again, and the stains and odors keep multiplying. Your carpet also becomes a haven for the growth of mold (another allergy trigger) and bacteria.

What Can You Do?

The first step is to locate soiled areas and clean and deodorize them thoroughly. Cats and dogs are very different when they make a "mistake" indoors. Dogs will often squat or lift their legs to urinate or defecate on the floor or horizontal objects right in front of you. Cats are more cunning; they hide their misdeeds behind a sofa or chair, under the bed, or some other place that's known only to them.

If you smell an odor but can't see the stain, try a black light (available at Home Depot or from mail-order supply houses listed in the Resource Guide). Turn out all lights in the room before you turn on the black light; urine that is deposited on walls or sprayed onto carpets, floors, upholstery, and furniture will show as fluorescent greenish spots or drips.

Cleaning Wet Stains

For carpets and upholstery:

- Blot up (don't scrub) as much urine as possible with white paper towels or old terry towels. Keep using dry towels and repeating this step until the area is nearly dry. For carpets, press or stand on the towels a few seconds to help absorb the liquid. Dilute the stained area with distilled water and blot again until barely damp.

- Neutralize by spraying or pouring on an enzymatic product such as Urine-Off Odor & Stain Remover or Nature's Miracle Stain & Odor Remover, formulations designed specifically to penetrate deep into carpet fibers, absorb the odors, and remove the stains. Follow manufacturer's directions, testing the cleaner on a small area to be sure it doesn't stain. If a nonallergic family member is not available to do this job, wear a facial mask to keep from inhaling the fumes, and gloves to protect your hands. A second treatment may be necessary. Do not clean with vinegar, household cleaners, or ordinary carpet cleaners; these will simply cover up the smell for a few days at most.

For hard surfaces:

- Soak up the urine with paper towels and clean with an enzymatic cleaner, following package directions, and dry.

Cleaning Old, Dried-In Carpet Stains

- To remove heavy stains, consider renting a wet vac or extractor from your local hardware store to clean the carpet as thoroughly as possible. Steam cleaning is not recommended as the heat can permanently set the stain and odor by bonding urine proteins into the carpet fibers. Wear a protective mask and gloves.

- Once the area is clean, follow with an enzymatic pet stain and odor remover as instructed above. You may need to repeat this step on hard-to-remove stains and odors.

- If the urine staining is excessive, especially if it has been present for a long time and you are highly allergic, consider seeking the advice or services of a professional carpet cleaner or replacing the carpet entirely.

For more advice, check the website of the Humane Society of the United States (www.hsus.org) under "Removing Pet Stains and Odors." After urinating inappropriately at a spot indoors, a stubborn cat or dog may habitually return there, even if you have cleaned and deodorized. One of the most effective deterrents to make a previously soiled spot unusable is to change the behavioral function of the area; for example, since cats and dogs rarely soil their sleeping or eating places, try temporarily putting their bedding or food dishes there.

Cat Litter Boxes: Another Allergy Trigger

Your cat's litter box *must* be scooped and cleaned regularly, and should *not* be located near ducts that circulate heat or air throughout the house, or near areas that you regularly use, especially main activity rooms and bedrooms. Unscented litter is less irritating to allergy sufferers than brands with strongly scented perfumes, deodorizers, or other additives. The fine dust from traditional coarse-grained clay litter can also aggravate allergies. Better choices would be clumping litter (highly absorbent clay ground into finely textured sandy particles); silica pellets (also called litter pearls); or natural litters made from a variety of substances that come in pellet, flake, and granule form, like World's Best Cat Litter (made from corn and corncob) or Yesterday's News (made from recycled newspapers). Natural litters, in particular, are highly absorbent and soak up liquid like a natural sponge.

Scooping the litter box *at least once a day* is the most effective way to control odor. After scooping, add a little fresh litter to replace what was removed, and dispose of the soiled litter immediately. Whenever possible, have a nonallergic family member clean the box and change the litter; if you do it yourself, wear gloves and a protective mask. Always pour fresh litter into the box slowly, to keep dust from permeating the air. Although clumping, pelleted, and silica litter manufacturers recommend a complete litter change only once a month, allergy sufferers should change litter *every week*. At that time, scrub the litter box in hot water and a mild dishwashing solution; rinse thoroughly; and dry, preferably outdoors in the sun. Every other cleaning, disinfect with a solution of one-quarter cup of chlorine laundry bleach per gallon of warm water, rinse and dry thoroughly. Do not use strong household cleaners or ammonia; the latter will only heighten the urine odors.

More good news for allergy sufferers is that there are now self-cleaning litter boxes that do all the dirty work for you. LitterMaid and Petmate Purrforma Plus, for instance, are the most popular fully automatic high-tech systems. You fill the litter box with clumping litter, and after your cat uses it, a sensor determines that the cat has exited the box and signals an automatic sifting comb to rake through the box and scoop up the waste, which is then deposited into a sealed, airtight container. Allergy sufferers can be away all day and know that the litter box will be clean after every use.

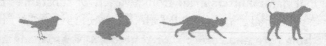

SIX

MINIMIZING BIRD ALLERGENS

All species of birds can produce allergic reactions in humans, and along with minimizing allergens on your bird, it is very important to keep its cage and all equipment scrupulously clean.

FEATHER DUST OR "POWDER": THE MAJOR BIRD ALLERGEN

The major bird allergen is derived from the powdery feather dust that coats their feathers. Studies show that allergy to feathers themselves is extremely rare. When birds preen themselves and flutter their wings, no matter how small they are, this fine feather dust is shaken off into the air to circulate throughout the house and collect in and around the cage. Feather dust from most of the larger species of parrots, especially from powder down birds—Cockatiels, Cockatoos, and African Grays—dramatically accumulates, especially in the room that houses the birdcage.

Bird droppings also cause sensitivities. Birds digest their food quickly and create a great deal of waste matter; it's been estimated that many birds have up to fifty eliminations per day! Cages that are not cleaned regularly are the perfect setting for the growth of many pathogens. In addition to feather dust, shed feathers, and feather particles, droppings and bits of spoiled food that have dried in the bottom of the cage are another source of dust and dust mites, and can be the breeding ground for mold spores, bacteria, viruses, and other organisms that aggravate allergies.

CHOICE AND PLACEMENT OF THE BIRDCAGE

Although birdcages can be quite elaborate, the most important feature for allergy sufferers is that they are easy to clean and disinfect. Since many birds love to climb and to chew, stainless steel cages are best because they are virtually indestructible. Birds are clever escape artists, so be sure cage latches are strong and secure. Different birds have vastly different spatial needs: be certain that the cage you choose is large enough for your bird (or birds) to stretch its wings without touching the sides and to move freely about between the perches without being obstructed in any way.

A cage with a removable floor tray will facilitate the cleaning of bird droppings each day. Line the cage floor with thick paper and tape it down to make cleaning easier. Pet birds should be housed in a room that can be adapted to minimize the spread of allergens (see chapter 12, "Allergen-Proofing Your Home"). Place the cage in an area where it can't be tipped over and away from direct sunlight, drafts, or sudden temperature changes, and fumes or other odors. Polytetrafluoroethylene gas emitted from overheated cookware coated with Teflon or Silverstone, and other nonstick pans, for instance, can be fatal to birds. Make sure, too, that any cats or dogs in the house cannot thrust their paws or noses into the cage, or otherwise gain access to it and injure the bird. Because of the amount of feather dust that can circulate in the air, *never* place the birdcage in the bedroom of an allergic person.

The area around the cage will also become soiled by food or

droppings. Many birds are very sloppy when they bathe and splash drops of water outside their cages. Stand your bird's cage on a washable surface, or protect your floors by placing it on a sheet of plastic. Avoid putting the birdcage in a room with carpeting. Installing a HEPA filter near the cage will also help to absorb and contain dust and dander allergens, and prevent them from circulating into other living spaces in your home, but do not place the filter too close to the cage, as doing so can cause the bird's skin to become dry, and drafts caused by the air circulating from the filter could make the bird sick.

CLEANING THE BIRDCAGE

Once a week, the bird's cage, the floor tray, and all accessories—perches, swings, ladders, mirrors, chains, and toys—need a routine washing. Whenever possible, the cleaning should be performed by someone other than the allergic person; otherwise the allergy sufferer should wear a protective face mask to avoid breathing in the feather dust. Put your bird into temporary accommodations such as a traveling cage or container with plenty of airholes while you clean.

A more thorough cleaning of the cage and tray is necessary about once a month. Use a firm brush to scrub everything in hot, soapy water; disinfect (experts recommend a twenty-minute soaking in a dilution of 4 ounces of chlorine bleach per gallon of water); then *rinse and dry thoroughly* before putting the bird back inside. Damp cages and trays can develop mold in and under them. If the perches are made of wood, it's smart to have an additional set. Wood takes a long time to dry and your bird's feet can become irritated by standing on a wet perch.

When cleaning the cage, use a damp sponge to wipe off any

feather dust on the bars and other washable surfaces, and a damp mop on floors to collect and hold the powder and keep it out of circulation. Dry-dusting will only circulate more bird allergens into the air; brooms are not only ineffective but actually intensify the problem. To keep feather dust and droppings from building up, drying out, and becoming airborne, change the papers on the cage bottom every day, as mold can easily grow on paper that becomes damp, triggering an allergy to molds. Rather than sweep the floor with a broom, have a nonallergic family member vacuum around the cage area to pick up any shed feathers, feather particles, or spilled seed husks that the bird has scattered about.

SANITARY PROCEDURES FOR DISPENSING FOOD AND WATER

See that fresh food and water, in clean containers, are available at all times. Pet stores sell plastic birdseed and water containers with special clamps that attach to the cage bars, as well as heavy earthenware dishes for serving fruits, greens, and other food. Always place the dishes away from the bird's perch or else they can become contaminated by droppings. Once a day, pick up all leftover seeds or other uneaten food. Wash all containers often in hot soapy water, rinse thoroughly, and dry before refilling.

CARE AND GROOMING

Birds usually keep themselves clean. Most will preen or clean their feathers (even very long tail feathers, when present) thoroughly several times a day by pulling them, one at a time, through their bills. Birds can artfully twist and contort themselves so that their bills reach all body parts except their heads, napes, and throats. In addition to grooming their plumage, birds also spread oil from their preening gland, located near the base of the tail, onto the feathers to help condition and lubricate them.

Physically and emotionally healthy birds spend a great deal of time preening. After these sessions (as well as after sleeping), birds will raise their feathers and shake them vigorously to align their plumage into proper order. Unfortunately for allergy sufferers, the twisting and rubbing movements of their heads and bills during preening, and the shaking of feathers, causes a great deal of feather dust to be released into the environment. Birds whose plumage contains powder down feathers produce significant amounts of dust when their feather tips disintegrate into a fine white powder, which is so minute that it quickly circulates throughout the house.

BATHING

Bathing is an extremely satisfying activity for birds and they enjoy baths or showers once or twice a week. In addition to keeping the skin and feathers in good condition, *bathing helps reduce the accumulation of feather dust.*

The best time to give your bird a bath is immediately before you clean the cage and re-paper the bottom, because the cage floor covering will get wet and need changing. (Remember: never let the floor covering become damp, otherwise mold can develop.) If it's cold outside, be sure the room is warm (at least 75° F or 23.8°C) and draft-free. It's a good idea to schedule the bath during the morning or afternoon, so that the feathers are totally dry before bedtime.

Canaries, Lovebirds, Budgies, and other small birds, as well as Mynas, love wriggling around in containers filled with water. Pet stores sell special bathing cups that clip onto the doorway of the birdcage, or you can simply place a shallow dish (to prevent drowning) on the cage bottom. Fill the container with tepid water, then let your bird go in and splash around as much as it wants. Most birds will hop out, shake their feathers, and plunge back in again, chirping with delight. Be sure to wash the bathing dish frequently.

Medium-sized and large parrots generally will not bathe themselves standing in a bowl of water. They do, however, enjoy a "shower," or a light misting of water from a spray bottle a couple of times a week, especially on warm days. Fill a clean spray bottle (never use a bottle that once contained cleaning agents or anything else unsafe) or plant mister with fresh, tepid (never cold) water. Set the nozzle for the finest mist possible. Hold the bottle about 12–15 inches away from the cage, and don't point it directly at the bird. Instead, spray into the air above the bird, letting the water drizzle down like raindrops. Some birds may be apprehensive of the sprayer to begin with, but in time they become so enthusiastic about their showers that they start vocalizing at the sight of the bottle, raise their feathers, and turn around on their perches to let the water reach them from all angles. Misting powder down birds daily with plain water will help keep excess powder from building up.

Your bird will be soaking wet after a bath, shower, or daily misting, and should be confined to a warm place until the feathers are totally dry, particularly if it's cold outside. Some medium-sized and large tame birds can be dried by a handheld electric dryer, but others may be frightened by the noise. Some birds may permit you to gently blot the excess moisture from their feathers with a towel. During the summer, let your bird occasionally enjoy a warm bath or shower outside.

CLEANSING THE FEATHERS WITH AN ALLERGY CLEANSING SOLUTION

Instead of a water bath or shower, another way for allergy sufferers to control the powder that scatters into the atmosphere is to lightly mist a pet allergy cleansing solution onto your bird's feathers once or twice a week, misting the solution away from the head and toward the tail. *Check the label recommendations of the product you choose to be sure it is safe to use on birds.* Allow the plumage to dry naturally or use a hair dryer. Keep the bird away from drafts until it is completely dry.

SEVEN

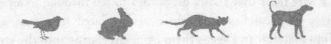

MINIMIZING RABBIT ALLERGENS

Rabbits belong to the order known as Lagomorpha, or harelike animals. There are more than sixty-five breeds and color varieties in the world, all descendants of European wild rabbits.

DANDER, SALIVA, AND URINE: THE MAJOR RABBIT ALLERGENS

All breeds of rabbits can cause allergic reactions in humans. The major rabbit allergens are derived from the dander or dead skin flakes they shed, the saliva that coats their fur when they self-groom, and their urine.

TIPS FOR HOUSING YOUR RABBIT

If your rabbit will live indoors, you may wish to keep it in a cage, or if it's housebroken, let the rabbit run free in the house during the day and confine it only at night. If your rabbit does run free, use an adjustable pet or baby gate to restrict territory to certain rooms to help prevent allergens from spreading throughout the house. *Never* allow the rabbit access to your bedroom or to upholstered furniture.

Basically, you need an easy-to-clean wire or wood-framed cage with a wire floor that allows droppings to fall through to a pull-out tray that catches any debris, accumulated hair, hay, and bedding material and keeps them from circulating into the environment. These cages are available from pet stores, farm supply stores, and rabbit supply companies. The size of the cage depends on how much time your rabbit spends inside it; the more time, the larger the cage should be. Cages that open from the side are preferable to those that open from the top. An experienced supply dealer can point out all the features of the different rabbit cage and door styles, and help you choose the right habitat and accessories.

One important feature to consider: you'll notice that cages are available in many different gauges of wire. Make sure the floor of your cage is made of approximately half inch or *slightly* larger welded wire, small enough to support the rabbit's feet, but large enough to allow droppings to pass through to the tray underneath. Rabbits can get their feet caught in larger wire and break or dislocate a hind leg. An optional urine guard, a metal strip that attaches around the inside base of the cage, will help the rabbit's urine flow into the cage bottom and not splash outside. Instead of lining the pull-out tray with straw (which can exacerbate allergies), aspen shavings, small animal cage litter, or cat litter made from corn or wheat all work well in the cage bottom; they are absorbent, keep odors down, and have low dust levels.

USING A LITTER BOX

Rabbits usually prefer to urinate and defecate in one corner of their cage or hutch and will readily use a litter box. Rabbit droppings don't smell as foul as cat feces, so if you place the box in the corner of the cage your rabbit chooses for a bathroom and scoop it out every day, the cage should stay odor free. Basic rectangular plastic cat trays (without lids) are fine for rabbits. Rabbits often chew their litter, so make sure the type you use is nontoxic if ingested. Critter Litter Potty Training Pearls or cat litter made from recycled newspapers in pellets or small pieces are good choices, because they are dust-free, hypoallergenic, superabsorbent, nontoxic, and environmentally friendly (and they can be flushed down the toilet in small quantities). Do not use litters made from cedar shavings or other aromatic soft woods, like pine, because they release hydrocarbons that can exacerbate asthma in rabbits and humans. Remove and dispose of soiled litter immediately. Change the litter completely at the same time that you clean and re-bed the entire cage.

Rabbits that are allowed to run free will instinctively select one special corner of a room to use as a bathroom. Place the litter box there, on newspapers to protect the floor if it isn't easy to clean. If an accident occurs, use an enzymatic cleaning product designed to remove pet stains and odors, carefully following the manufacturer's directions.

SANITARY PROCEDURES FOR DISPENSING FOOD AND WATER

Rabbits usually eat a varied diet consisting of commercial rabbit pellets (sold at pet stores), plus greens and vegetables. Heavy earthenware crocks that can't be turned over are best for greens and vegetables, while food hoppers or self-feeders work well for bite-sized pellets (some clip to the wall of the cage and can be filled from the outside). Choose a hopper or feeder that has a screened, not solid, bottom to allow the fine dust from the food to pass through and not build up. Place feeding dishes close to the door of the cage, *as far away as possible from the rabbit's toilet area.* Feed only as much as will be eaten by the next feeding time, otherwise some rabbits will soil their food by urinating or defecating in their dishes. Since water can quickly become dirty and contaminated, a gravity-fill automatic water bottle with stainless steel sipping tube that attaches to the cage is preferable.

Rabbits also need roughage in their diet. High-quality legume, timothy, or oat hay satisfies a rabbit's desire to chew and aids in their digestion. Pet stores stock hay cubes or hay packed in small bags. Small tubs or wire racks that attach to the inside of the cage prevent food from becoming soiled or contaminated before eating. Add just enough hay to the rack to last until the next day and store the remainder in a lidded container outside, not in the house. Cover the top of the rack to keep your rabbit from hopping inside and getting trapped or soiling the hay.

Be aware that the dust and pollen from hay can exacerbate allergies. Misting hay with water can help to reduce dust. Be sure to clean hay tubs, hoppers, crockery dishes, and water dispensers daily in warm, sudsy water and rinse thoroughly. Wear a protective mask when handling hay and cleaning to keep from inhaling allergens.

CLEANING THE CAGE

Every day, dampen a cloth (or use a disposable cage wipe, available at pet stores) and wipe the cage bars to remove any dander, shed hair, urine, or dried droppings. If you choose to line the bottom tray with papers, change everything daily to keep dried urine and droppings from building up. Once a week, the cage, floor tray, accessories, and toys should be washed in warm, soapy water, rinsed thoroughly, and dried completely, as mold can develop if they are left damp. After cleaning, vacuum around the cage area to pick up any debris that has scattered about.

A more thorough cleaning of the cage and tray is necessary once a month. Use a firm brush to scrub everything in hot soapy water, rinse, and then disinfect in a solution made by mixing 4 ounces of household bleach per gallon of water. Rinse thoroughly again, and dry the cage completely before putting your rabbit back inside. Have a nonallergic family member do the cleaning or wear a protective mask.

CARE AND GROOMING

Rabbits are fastidiously clean animals. Unfortunately for allergy sufferers, they groom themselves meticulously by licking their fur. Like cats, each lick of a rabbit's tongue deposits saliva on the fur which, when dry, flakes off and becomes airborne to circulate throughout the house. The many different rabbit breeds come in different coat types: short-haired, plush, and long-haired (such as the Jersey Wooly and Angora). Brushing them at least twice a week with a soft bristle or wire slicker brush (depending on coat type) removes loose hair, dander, and dust, particularly when they are shedding. Another alternative is to use a grooming glove with textured dots that grabs and pulls out loose hair. Use a metal comb to gently tease out tangles on the longhairs. Angora rabbits have coats that grow continuously and they need to have their hair trimmed short on a regular basis (a professional groomer can do this) so that it doesn't get as matted, dirty, or loaded with allergens, and is easier to manage.

Rabbits shed hair three or four times a year in alternating

patterns—one shed will be light, the next shed will be heavy—which usually start at the head and gradually extend to the tail. In the case of Angoras, you can anticipate the start of a shedding period when you find the hair becoming more matted than usual, and when there is more loose hair in your comb after grooming.

In addition to helping alleviate allergens, brushing rabbits with a fine-wire slicker brush will help to prevent the formation of hairballs, a potentially serious condition in rabbits. During their normal self-grooming procedure, rabbits will naturally ingest loose dead hair. Unlike cats, who can regurgitate hairballs, rabbits cannot vomit, and they can swallow so much loose fur, especially during heavy periods, that a life-threatening hairball may form in the digestive tract. This condition, known as "wool block," can become serious and require veterinary treatment. Hairball lubricants or laxatives such as those used on cats can help prevent hairballs. Feeding fresh pineapple juice or pineapple chunks which contain the enzyme papain may also help. Check with your veterinarian for more information about rabbit health care.

CLEANING THE HAIR

Rabbits do *not* need to be bathed; in fact, immersing them in water can be very stressful to them. A rabbit should *only* be bathed if it has fleas, if it becomes soiled from having diarrhea, or if its anal area is caked with fecal matter. Try spot cleaning any soiled areas first by wiping with a washcloth and warm water. Bathe only as a last resort, following instructions found in chapter 8, "Minimizing Rodent Allergens." Dry the rabbit as soon as possible with a towel or hair dryer and keep it in a warm location until the hair is dry.

To remove dander, saliva, and urine allergens, once a week, moisten a washcloth with a pet allergy cleansing solution and wipe over the fur, first with and then against the lay of the hair. Check the label recommendations of the product you choose to be sure it is safe to use on rabbits. Let the product remain on the fur, blot it dry with a towel, and keep the rabbit in a warm, draft-free area until completely dry. Some rabbits enjoy being dried by a hair dryer, but others may be frightened by the noise.

EIGHT

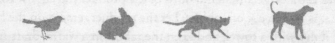

MINIMIZING RODENT ALLERGENS
Gerbils, Guinea Pigs, Hamsters, Chinchillas, Mice, and Rats

Rodents have become increasingly popular housepets, of both adults and children. They make ideal first-time pets for children and help them to develop humane instincts and empathy for other living creatures.

URINE, DANDER, AND SALIVA: THE MAJOR RODENT ALLERGENS

Even though most rodents are caged, their major allergens are derived from urine, saliva, and dander. Studies indicate that urine from guinea pigs, hamsters, mice, rats, and chinchillas contains potent allergens that can trigger reactions. In the case of guinea pigs and gerbils, additional allergens from dander and saliva also have been identified.

HOUSING

Choosing the proper habitat will increase your enjoyment of your rodent, as well as play an important role in its health and your allergies. Basically you will need: (a) a secure, easy-to-clean wire cage with a solid metal or plastic bottom floor, as most rodents have no fur on the bottoms of their feet to protect them from getting caught in wire; (b) a washable, see-through plastic habitat with tunnels and rooms; or (c) a glass or acrylic aquarium tank with a cover. As with rabbits, access from the cage side is preferable to access from the top. The cage type and size will depend on the type and number of rodents you want to house, but you should provide plenty of room for them to move around.

Your pet supplies dealer can recommend the right housing; he can also show you how to set up and equip your rodent's habitat with the proper tunnels, ramps, mazes, exercise wheels, toys, bedding, floor mats, and other necessities appropriate for each small animal. Rodents also like to retreat into little sleeping boxes, so make sure your rodent has its own special place in which to hide. You'll also need to cover the cage floor with nontoxic, absorbent, biodegradable, dust-free material as nesting material for your rodent to burrow in for warmth. Straw is not a good choice for allergy sufferers as it can contain dust, mold, and pollen that may exacerbate your allergies. Instead, choose small animal cage litter or bedding such as Kaytee Kay-Kob (natural corncob), Green Pet Products Clean-N-Comfy Litter Bedding, softwood shavings (aspen shavings in particular, which contain no aromatic oils), or any of the cat litters made from whole kernel corn (World's Best Cat Litter), wheat (Swheat Scoop), or recycled paper pellets (Yesterday's News). Never use cedar shavings as they can cause respiratory problems in some rodents.

Rodents cannot be housebroken but they do tend to select the same small areas of their cages to eliminate, making it easier for you to remove smelly clumps. Laying a glass jar on its side in the cage (with some shavings inside) often encourages rodents to use it as a "litter jar." Empty the jar daily, wash with hot sudsy water, and rinse well.

Placement of the cage is important. Rodents are highly susceptible to chilling and overheating; keep the cage in a well-ventilated room, away from drafts, air-conditioning, vents, radiators, or windows that are hit by direct sunlight. Also ensure that other pets, specifically cats or dogs, cannot jab their paws or noses into the cage or otherwise gain access to it. While many rodent owners don't allow their pets to run around on the floors, they do often allow them access to couches, tabletops, beds, and other furniture. Unfortunately, allergy sufferers should consider this a no-no.

SANITARY PROCEDURES FOR DISPENSING FOOD AND WATER

Rodents eat grass hay, alfalfa, seeds, and pelleted food supplemented with fresh fruit and vegetables. You can buy small bundles of premium-quality timothy hay and alfalfa at your local pet store. Feeding racks (for hay) that attach to the cage and heavy earthenware dishes are recommended because they can't be tipped over. Fill the hay racks outside and store the hay outside as well, not in the house. *Water in a bowl can become contaminated within minutes by spilled food, urine, and feces.* A gravity-fill automatic water bottle with a stainless steel sipping tube that attaches to the cage is more sanitary.

Rodents, especially guinea pigs, can be quite messy, scattering food about the cage, defecating in feeding bowls, and spitting food back into water bottles. Pick up all spilled food promptly, otherwise it will become contaminated by urine, fecal matter, or soiled bedding. Always wash dishes and water bottles before refilling them. Scrub the water dispenser with a bottle brush to prevent algae and bacteria from developing inside. Replace bottles that develop a scum or film.

CLEANING THE CAGE

It's extremely important to keep your cage or habitat clean because rodent urine is not only unpleasant smelling but also, and more importantly, a primary source of allergens. Although rodents are naturally clean in the wild, when they are confined to a cage or habitat, urine and fecal matter accumulate quickly and cause a strong odor. In addition, certain rodents, particularly sexually mature males, emit strong-smelling odors from their scent glands. These strong-smelling odors may trigger allergies as well.

Urine-soaked bedding is a potent allergy trigger. It dries in the bedding material and is then circulated into the air when pets scramble in their cage or when the soiled bedding is removed during cleaning. Always keep bedding dry to prevent odors and fungus from developing.

Ask your pet supplies dealer to recommend a deodorizing product that can be added daily to the cage bedding. Allergy sufferers especially need to prevent urine odors that result from chemicals emitted from rodent urine—mouse urine is especially high in ammonia content. Male urine smells the strongest, but females can also excrete pungent urine. If urine odor is not eliminated during the cleaning process, it will remain and become stronger over time. Enzymatic formulations that break down urine and fecal matter can help neutralize odors.

Frequent cage cleaning will help to reduce the amount of urine, dander, and salivary proteins which often trigger allergies in sensitive individuals. Every day, wipe off the cage bars with a damp cloth or a disposable cage wipe (available at pet stores). Dry-dusting will only direct more allergens into the air. Remove any damp clumps of bedding in the cage corners that have been used as a bathroom with an old spoon or tiny scoop, and refresh the cage by adding new fill.

Once a week, the cage or habitat, floor tray, tubes, modules, toys, exercise wheels, and other accessories need to be washed in hot soapy water, rinsed thoroughly, and dried, preferably by a nonallergic family member. Wear a protective facial mask if that's not possible. Many habitat accessories are dishwasher safe. Add fresh bedding when the cage is dry. If you have multiple rodents or detect a urine or ammonia odor, replace the bedding more often.

Once a month, in addition to washing the cage, disinfect by soaking it in a solution of 4 ounces of chlorine bleach per gallon of water. Rinse thoroughly and dry completely before adding fresh bedding and nesting material and putting the pet back inside. Do not use strong household cleaners or disinfectants as some can be toxic to rodents. During the cleaning and drying, of course, place your pet in a separate cage or well-ventilated box to keep it safe. Always wash your hands and arms after handling your rodent.

RODENT GROOMING

Here are some specific grooming suggestions to help reduce allergens. These focus on brushing, combing, and cleaning; check with your veterinarian about other health care requirements.

- *Gerbils* need little grooming from their owners. They keep themselves and each other scrupulously clean with their tongues, teeth, and paws. Being desert animals, native to arid regions of northeastern China and eastern Mongolia, they excrete very little urine and have hardly any odor. Brush them occasionally with a small bristle brush or soft toothbrush to remove dander, their primary allergen.

- *Guinea pigs* or *cavies* require grooming between once and several times a week, depending on the breed. Like cats, they are fastidious cleaners, grooming themselves with their tongues, teeth, and paws. Guinea pigs have a single-hair coat that comes in various lengths and textures and requires different maintenance to reduce allergens.

1. Short-haired cavies have soft and smooth hair that lies close to the skin. Brush them from head to tail, in the direction that the hair grows, with a small soft bristle brush to remove loose hair and dander.

2. Abyssinian cavies have medium-stiff hair, about 2 inches long, that stands outward from the body to form a series of rosettes and ridges. Brush them with a small, fine-wire slicker, stroking the brush upward and outward.

3. Peruvians have long, soft hair with a forelock that falls over their faces, making it difficult at times to tell the front end from the rear. The long hair grows continually (up to 20 inches if not cut) and requires lots of attention and grooming, otherwise it quickly becomes tangled and urine, dander, and salivary secretions will become trapped in the mats. Brush them at least twice a week with a bristle or slicker brush and then comb the hair from the skin outward to keep it from matting. Allergy sufferers should have

their Peruvians' hair trimmed to floor length or even shorter to make them easier to keep clean and prevent the coat from soaking up urine.

4. Teddies (or teddy bears) have short, kinky wire coats that are non-matting, but tend to collect dust, dirt, and shavings. Texels (long-haired teddies) have an identical kinky wire coat, but it is longer in length. Brush each with a fine-wire slicker brush at least twice a week.

- *Hamsters* spend a great deal of their waking time thoroughly grooming themselves with their tongues, teeth, and paws to keep their fur in good condition. Short-haired hamsters need to be brushed only occasionally, while long-haired types need more frequent grooming with a small bristle brush or soft toothbrush to keep the cage free of contaminated excess hair.

- *Chinchillas* have more elaborate grooming requirements than gerbils, guinea pigs, and hamsters. Native to the arid mountainous regions of Peru, Chile, and Bolivia, they are exceptional in that they like to "bathe" every day in a fine cindery dust or sand to maintain and condition their soft pearly gray fur to keep it from becoming oily. Special chinchilla bath dust/sand is available at pet stores.

  Schedule a dust bath at the same time each day, preferably in the evening. The "bathtub" should be a solid, chew-proof container (such as a ceramic or glass bowl) large and sturdy enough for your chinchilla to move around in without turning over. *Wear a dust mask!*

Pour about an inch or two of bath dust in the bottom of the bowl and place it inside the cage on top of several layers of paper towels. Your chinchilla will jump in immediately and clean its fur by rolling around continuously for about 15–20 minutes.

During the bathing and rolling process, of course, the chinchilla will spread the dust in and around its cage. To reduce the amount of dust that escapes into the air, remove the container *immediately* after the bath, discard the paper towels, and wipe any dusty surfaces on and around the cage with a dampened cloth or sponge.

A chinchilla's fine, silky hair needs to be brushed occasionally with a soft toothbrush or small bristle brush, and combed to remove the dead fur and dust. Chinchillas constantly shed their hair and clumps of dead hair can collect in the corners of the cage. Combing a chinchilla before letting it roll in the dust bath will keep the loose, shed hair from accumulating in the cage.

- *Mice* and *rats* are extremely fastidious. They groom themselves and each other in a colony without any help from their owners. To help remove dead fur, though, use a small brush or toothbrush with soft bristles and brush, stroking with the lay of the hair, from head to tail.

CLEANSING RODENTS

With the exception of chinchillas, who dislike being wet, all other rodents mentioned in this section need a bath *only* if they smell bad or if their rear ends are sticky with urine or caked with feces. Pet stores sell instant rodent shampoos that you wipe on and do not rinse off. These loosen dirt, dissolve oils, and leave the pet smelling fresh without conventional bathing.

When a bath is necessary, use a mild, tearless shampoo formulated for cats and kittens. Some rodents have stronger body odor than others, so you may want to use a special rodent deodorant shampoo, such as Superpet Squeaky Clean Critter Shampoo. Fill a bathroom sink or plastic dishpan with a little warm water and shampoo; put your pet inside and gently pour small cupfuls over the body. Wash the pet, rinse the fur thoroughly, then blot it dry with a towel. Keep the pet in a warm, draft-free area. Be sure it is completely dry before returning to its cage or habitat, as rodents are highly susceptible to chilling.

You can also cleanse the urine, saliva, and dander allergens from small furry pets once a week by moistening a washcloth with a pet allergy relief solution or using a pet allergy wipe. *Check the label recommendations on the product you choose to be sure it is safe to use on rodents.* Rub over the fur with and against the growth. Blot dry with a towel; keep the pet warm until it is completely dry. A weekly pet allergy cleansing will also keep the animal clean and sweet smelling. Wash your hands and arms immediately after handling your rodent.

NINE

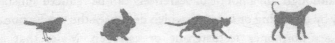

MINIMIZING FERRET ALLERGENS

Ferrets are Mustelids that belong to the same family as skunks, minks, weasels, badgers, and otters. They are fastidious, intelligent, affectionate, quiet, and gentle creatures that are incredibly social.

FERRET ALLERGENS: URINE, DANDER, AND SEBACEOUS GLAND SECRETIONS

Although there has been limited formal testing to determine ferret allergens, they are likely derived from urine, dander, and secretions from the sebaceous skin glands.

FERRETS AND MUSKY ODORS

Allergy sufferers should know that the ferret's oily sebaceous skin glands (spread around the face and body) and well-developed anal scent glands secrete musk, giving them a very strong odor which many people find offensive. These pungent secretions, stronger in intact adult males, can also cause the fur to feel greasy and assume a yellow cast. *Musky ferret odors can be irritating to allergy sufferers.* Getting rid of the musk odor entirely is not possible, although the amount of secretions can be reduced substantially by neutering or spaying, which decreases the production of the sex hormones testosterone or estrogen. Males that are neutered may still produce a slight odor, but females that are spayed seldom produce any odor. De-scenting, a controversial medical procedure to remove the scent glands near the tail, is usually not necessary.

HOUSING YOUR FERRET

Ferrets need lots of exercise and playtime, and should not be isolated in a cage for long periods of time, so your ferret will occasionally need to run free in the house. It is important, however, to restrict its territory to certain rooms to help prevent allergens from spreading. *Never* allow your ferret access to your bedroom or upholstered furniture.

Basically, ferrets are best housed in easy-to-clean wire cages with secure latches, as they are clever escape artists. No part of the cage should be made of wood; it soaks up urine and the odor is impossible to remove. Cages should be roomy—at least 30–36 inches long, 18 inches wide, and 18 inches high—to provide separate areas for eating, sleeping, and discharging urine and feces. Because ferrets love to climb, multiple-level "ferret condos" (cages with two or three stories) are ideal and adding hammocks will help prevent falls from the top level. Cover the bottom of the cage with a washable rug because a ferret's paws are not designed to walk on wire floors.

Ferrets often sleep the majority of the day, and they don't enjoy sleeping in the open. Therefore, you'll need to make a little "bedroom" area where they can nest. Small cardboard boxes or baskets and ferret sleeping bags or snuggle tubes make good choices. Bedding material can consist of Kaytee Kay-Kob Bedding & Litter (natural corncob), Green Pet Products Clean-N-Comfy, shredded white paper, or an old washable T-shirt. Sawdust or cedar chips should not be used for bedding because they represent a respiratory risk to ferrets and aggravate your allergies as well. Wood chips, too, will quickly absorb urine, feces, and musk odors but make your allergies worse.

Place the cage in a cool area away from direct sunlight; ferrets cannot tolerate temperatures above 90° F (30° C) because they have underdeveloped sweat glands.

USING A LITTER BOX

Ferrets like to relieve themselves in the same place every time. Because they are intelligent, they can be trained to use a litter box. Small cat litter pans are fine, as are plastic dishpans. Critter Litter Potty Training Pearls (for ferrets and small animals) or cat litters made from recycled newspapers in the form of pellets or small pieces are an excellent choice because they are dust-free, nonallergenic, nontoxic, superabsorbent, and environmentally friendly (they can be flushed down the toilet in small quantities). Clay litters are not recommended for ferrets, especially the clumping varieties, as sniffing and inhaling the litter or dragging their bottoms across it can cause the small granules to clump inside their noses or rectums and cause problems. As mentioned in chapter 7, litters made of cedar shavings and other aromatic softwoods are also not recommended, because they release volatile hydrocarbons that affect those animals living within them.

Place the litter box in a corner of the cage and scoop it daily to minimize odors. Change the litter completely at the same time you clean the cage and accessories.

CLEANING THE CAGE AND BEDDING

It's extremely important to keep your ferret's cage and bedding clean, not only to minimize allergens but also to help reduce some of the musky odor. Every day wipe off the cage bars with a damp cloth or deodorizing cage wipe (available at pet stores). Dry-dusting will only direct more allergens into the air. Frequent changing or laundering of the bedding will also help prevent musk oils from building up.

Once a week (twice a week during spring and fall shedding seasons), the cage should be washed in hot soapy water, rinsed thoroughly and dried, preferably by a nonallergic family member. Wear a protective facial mask if that's not possible. Add fresh nesting material when the cage is dry. Once a month, in addition to washing the cage, disinfect it by soaking in a solution of 4 ounces of chlorine bleach per gallon of water, then rinse and dry it thoroughly before adding clean bedding and nesting materials. Do not use strong household cleaners or disinfectants as some can be toxic to ferrets. Always wash your hands and arms after handling your ferret.

SANITARY PROCEDURES FOR DISPENSING FOOD AND WATER

To prevent food spillage, use a heavy, shallow earthenware bowl (placed away from the litter pan) that can't be tipped over. Give water via a bottle with a stainless steel sipping tube that attaches to the side of the cage. Wash the feeding dish and water bottle daily.

GROOMING

Ferrets have soft, dense double coats: a soft and dense undercoat that acts as insulation, and an outer coat of longer guard hairs. They shed their fur twice a year to produce a soft, lightweight spring/summer coat and a thicker, denser fall/winter coat. Hair shedding can be especially dramatic in the spring. Brush the fur (with a soft bristle brush) at least once a week to remove all loose hair that is contaminated with dander, sebaceous skin gland, and urinary secretions. During shedding periods, the fur needs to be brushed every day. If your ferret is shedding excessively, you may want to temporarily "pluck" or pull out patches of loose dead hair. Stop, though, if the hair doesn't come out easily; it's just not ready to be plucked.

Like rabbits, ferrets do lick themselves on occasion and swallow loose hair in the process, which can form into hairballs in the stomach. This can be especially dangerous during the spring and fall shedding periods because not all ferrets regurgitate their hairballs. Ask your veterinarian or pet supplies dealer about laxative treatments to prevent hairballs. As plenty of dead hair also collects in the bedding during shedding periods, change it more often than usual at this time.

Ferret hair often smells muskier during spring and fall shedding seasons. *Never* spray your ferret's coat with colognes or other scented human products in an attempt to mask odors, as this can cause respiratory problems for both you and your ferret. Your pet supplies dealer can recommend safe products that are formulated for ferret coats. Wash your hands immediately after grooming.

BATHING AND CLEANSING YOUR FERRET

Even if your ferret has been neutered or spayed, it may still emit a little musky odor and the coat may feel greasy. Bathing is necessary, but no more than two to three times per month. Over-bathing can dry out the skin and hair; after a bath the skin glands tend to become overproductive in an effort to replace the oils that washed off. This can make a ferret smell worse for a few days afterward. Pet stores stock special ferret shampoos that will cleanse the hair and control musky odors. Ferret Sheen, for instance, a deodorizing shampoo, is specially formulated to eliminate ferret odors. Tearless cat shampoos are also safe for ferrets.

Carefully shampoo your ferret in warm water in the sink or in a small plastic dishpan. Fill the basin or dishpan with about 2 inches of warm water before placing your ferret inside. Add a little shampoo to the water and swirl it around with your fingers to make lather. Put the ferret in the water, holding it gently but securely, and shampoo starting at the head and working down to the tail. Rinse thoroughly to remove all traces of suds. Blot the hair with a towel and keep your ferret in a warm, draft-free room until it is completely dry. Wash your hands immediately after.

To control dander and sebaceous and urinary gland secretions, you can also use an allergy relief solution for pets once a week. Moisten a washcloth with the product and rub your ferret's fur in both directions, with and against the hair growth. Do not rinse the product off the coat, and dry as usual.

TEN

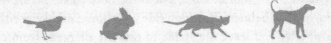

MINIMIZING HORSE ALLERGENS

Horses are highly allergenic animals, dander and urine being the most important sources of their allergens. As mentioned in chapter 3, practically everything associated with horses and their environment can cause allergic reactions: the animals themselves; the horsy odor produced when they sweat; their manure; the hay, oats, and other grains they eat; the mold spores growing in damp hay in their barns and stables; and even the saddles, harnesses, and bridles they wear. If you are allergic and still love horses and riding, the best advice is to avoid grooming them yourself and spending time *in* their barns and stables, especially during humid weather. Have someone else tack the horse; do your riding away from the stables; wipe down your tack after every ride; wash your hands, arms, and face thoroughly as soon as you leave the stable or barn; and change your clothing immediately afterward; do not bring riding attire, boots, or other accessories into your home.

HOW TO REDUCE HORSE ALLERGENS

The best way to minimize allergens consists of cleaning, both the horse and the barn. If you must do the cleaning yourself, wear rubber gloves, a face mask, and goggles to protect you from contact with dander and dust before you groom, tack, or clean the barn, stable, or ground. Also, put on a head scarf before you groom, or your helmet before you ride your horse, and keep either on until after you leave the stable to prevent allergens from collecting in your hair and ending up on your pillow.

A thorough daily brushing of the horse is a good way to start. This is especially important in the spring when horses are shedding their winter coats. Try not to do this in your horse's stall; providing it is warm, grooming outside in the open air is preferable. Use a rubber currycomb (an oval or circular "comb" with soft rubber teeth) or stiff bristle brush. Start at the top of the neck and work down the body, stroking in circular motions to loosen as much dead hair, dander, dirt, and mud as possible. Do not curry the legs. Pick up each foot; use a hoof pick (sold at tack shops) to remove any caked mud, and then use the stiff bristle brush to clean the soles and remove small particles that may be stuck in between. Then repeat these steps on the opposite side. Do not use the curry on your horse's face.

Investing in a horse vacuum (available at tack shops) or a wet/dry vacuum from a hardware store is helpful. After the currying loosens the dead hair and dander from the coat, turn on the vacuum and hold the nozzle close to the horse's body to lift off the dander and dust and keep it from becoming airborne and flying around the barn. In place of a horse vacuum, use a stiff bristle brush (everywhere but the face), stroking in the direction of the hair growth, to remove all the dirt that the currying loosens. Use this brush on the legs. Follow with a medium-bristled body brush to smooth down the hair. Use a mane-and-tail comb (a plastic comb with wide teeth that won't break the hairs) followed by the brush to gently go through the horse's mane and tail. Using a detangling lotion or spray on the mane or tail once or twice weekly makes it easy for the comb and brush to pass through the long hair. Finish by wiping over the coat with a towel to bring out the shine.

BATHING HELPS

This is a very brief description of how to bathe a horse. Some excellent books and websites giving more detailed advice are recommended in the Resource Guide. Use a shampoo that is pH balanced for horses, and mix it with warm water in a bucket. Begin by wetting the horse all over down to the skin (except for the head) with warm water from a hose. Be sure to lift the tail and wet the area around and under the anus and down between the hind legs and then wet the tail itself.

Apply the shampoo with a giant-sized sponge, working methodically up the front legs, over the shoulders, the neck and mane, down the back, down the flanks and hind legs, under the body and between the legs, then dunk the tail into the bucket. Using a rubber currycomb or rubber grooming mitt in a circular motion, work in the sudsy water to dislodge the loose hair, dander, and dirt. Use your fingers to shampoo the longer mane and tail hair, working the suds through the longer hair down to the skin. Keep adding shampoo and additional water to maintain enough suds. If the horse is really dirty, hose the suds off and shampoo a second time.

Horses usually don't enjoy having their heads washed, and it's a good idea to have another bucket ready in which you have mixed a little less shampoo with water. Wash the face and head gently. Use a bucket of clean water and fresh sponge (wringing it out often) to rinse off the suds.

When you have finished, use the hose to rinse the horse in the reverse order of how you wetted and soaped him. Use the hose (not on the face) or a fresh bucket of warm water and a clean sponge to thoroughly rinse the horse over and over until clear water runs off. Leaving a soapy residue can lead to itching and irritation. Don't forget to rinse under the stomach. Lift the tail and rinse underneath, then give the longer tail hair a thorough rinsing. When you have finished rinsing, you may want to apply a product such as Dander-Off for Horses (use according to directions).

Dry the head with a clean terry towel, blotting away any remaining moisture around the eyes and ears. Take a clean wrung-out sponge and wipe the excess moisture from the body and legs, squeezing it out frequently. A sweat scraper will also remove excess water, but avoid using the scraper on the legs as it's too uncomfortable for the horse. Finish by drying the body and legs with towels to give your horse a final polish.

CONCLUSION

Anything that is used on a horse—blankets, saddle pads, leg bandages, and tack—must be clean. Vacuum the feed bins, blankets, and tack trunks several times a week. To prevent mold from growing on the saddle in warm weather, wipe it occasionally with a cloth dampened with vinegar, before you condition the leather. In *Horse-Sense: The Newsletter of Holistic Horsemanship*, Jessica Jahiel (see Resources) suggests that any serious rider, especially one who is allergic, should install a washer and dryer in the tack room if they can. "It's very convenient," she writes, "to be able to drop saddle pads, bandages, etc. in the washing machine right there in the barn, instead of carrying them into the house while spreading dust and hair every step of the way." Ask your allergist to recommend antihistamines and other medications to take before riding or visiting the barn, or an immunization to decrease your sensitivity to horse allergens.

Note: many people who are allergic find that they are able to ride and handle Curly horses, perhaps because their coats are soft and form into ringlets, similar to Poodle hair. For more information, log on to the Internet and search under "Curly horses."

ELEVEN

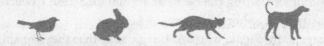

OTHER SUBSTANCES THAT MAKE PET ALLERGIES WORSE

If you are sensitive to pet allergens, you are probably allergic to other airborne nonanimal sources found in and around your home. Reducing or eliminating these from your environment will greatly help to lower your allergic threshold and make living with your pet more comfortable.

PERENNIAL ALLERGIC RHINITIS

If airborne allergies are a constant problem, then you are most likely suffering from perennial allergic rhinitis. As its name implies, perennial allergic rhinitis is a year-round condition caused (in addition to pet allergens) by sensitivities to a range of indoor allergens such as dust mites; cockroaches; molds and mildew; perfumes; household cleaners, chemicals, and soaps; pesticide sprays; tobacco smoke; pungent cooking odors; combustion pollutants (gas ranges and ovens, space heaters, fireplaces); and more. People who are allergic to pets are generally not aware of the significant role these other allergens, particularly dust mites, play in their sensitivities.

DUST MITES

Dust mites are *the major indoor allergen.* About 15 to 20 million Americans are allergic to dust mites. They are microscopic creatures that have been sharing our environment for centuries. In most homes with dust mites, the most prevalent are *Dermatophagoides farinae* and *Dermatophagoides pteronyssinus,* Latin names meaning "skin eaters," and that is exactly what they are. They feed primarily on dead skin flakes that are regularly shed from humans and animals.

Dust mites are invisible to the naked eye. They live in carpets (especially those with long or loose pile), overstuffed furniture, dusty bookcases, clothing and other items made from textured fabrics, and even stuffed toys, but especially in warm and humid places like pillows, mattresses, blankets, and comforters where your skin scales collect and serve as food sources. According to Larry Arlian, Ph.D., professor of biological sciences at the School of Medicine, Wright State University in Dayton, Ohio, in areas in a home where they are most prevalent, one teaspoon of house dust might contain between 500 and 1,000 mites!

Dust mite levels are at their highest in the summer and early fall, especially when the humidity is above 50 percent. Since they do not drink water, but absorb moisture from the environment and the air, they don't survive well in low humidity, dry climates, or at high altitudes. Studies indicate that in humid north- and southeastern cities like Cleveland, Memphis, or Houston, nearly all homes are dust mite positive, as compared to less than 10 percent of homes in drier and higher elevated climates like Denver.

The allergic potential of dust mites is not actually caused by the mites themselves, but by the powerful proteins contained in their fecal matter, decomposing body parts, and secretions. When these allergens dry out, they become airborne as soon as you shake your bedding, fluff a pillow, or walk across a rug. When inhaled, they stick to the moist lining of the nose where they can trigger an almost immediate allergic or asthmatic reaction. There is a strong correlation between these pesky critters and asthma that babies and children are especially vulnerable to.

Dust mites can live almost anywhere in your house, but are most often found in the bedroom, where millions of them live in your pillows, mattresses, sheets, and blankets. There they hatch, eat, defecate, and lay eggs. Your bed is their palace. The heat of your body, the moisture your body emits, and the food of your dead skin cells is the equivalent of a dust mite luxury spa—extraordinary ambience, luxurious accommodations, and outstanding cuisine! If you'd like to see what live dust mites actually look like in action, log on to www.de-mite.com. Suggestions for reducing their allergens are found in chapter 12, "Allergen-Proofing Your Home," a room-by-room guide to making your house as allergen-free as possible.

COCKROACHES

About 10 million Americans are allergic to cockroaches. Of five common species, the German and Brownbanded varieties are most common indoors, especially in apartment buildings. Cockroaches are nocturnal creatures that prefer warm, dark, and narrow places, close to food and water. Adult German cockroaches, according to the University of California, can hide in a crack $\frac{1}{16}$ inch (1.6 mm) wide. They multiply rapidly; the eggs of a single female and her offspring can produce over 30,000 cockroaches in a year.

Like dust mites, their potential to cause allergies does not come from the cockroaches themselves, but by proteins of their fecal matter, saliva, cast skins, and decomposing body parts. Cockroach allergens are highest in kitchens, but can also be found in beds, bedding, overstuffed furniture, and carpets.

Studies have shown that cockroach allergens are an important cause of asthma, especially in children and people that live in urban areas. If you live in an apartment building—especially one that has restaurants or food shops on the ground floor—cockroach infestation can be extremely hard to eliminate without the help of a professional exterminator. Part of the problem, write Dr. William Berger and Debra Gordon in their book *Allergy & Asthma Relief* (see Resource Guide) is that cockroaches eat anything—food, grease, paper, cardboard, dirty clothes, each other's feces, and they are especially fond of beer! The key to cockroach management is sanitation and exclusion; the conditions that attract and support them must be changed.

Tips for Controlling Cockroaches

- The first step is elimination. You can enlist the services of a professional exterminator, or you can use sticky pheromone traps or insecticides. (Pheromones are natural body chemicals produced by living organisms that attract other members of the same species to them.) If you don't want to use anything that could be potentially toxic to your pet, try dusting areas where roaches are known to hide with boric acid powder. Providing it remains dry and undisturbed, boric acid powder is effective for long periods. A light dusting is sufficient. The powder clings to the roaches as they walk through it and they die within hours of ingesting it. Be sure to keep the powder away from areas where you prepare food.

- Clean your home thoroughly to eliminate all dead roaches.

- After cleaning, limit all avenues of access and hiding places. Seal cracks and holes in walls, floors, door and window screens, and other openings to the outside. Eliminating plumbing leaks is especially important since cockroaches are attracted to moisture.

- Clean kitchen cabinets regularly as well as under stoves, refrigerators, toasters, or toaster ovens where crumbs can accumulate.

- Clean kitchen surfaces regularly; remove spilled food or beverages promptly.

- Store all food in sealed glass or plastic containers.

- Vacuum floors to remove food and debris.

- Wash dishes and utensils immediately in hot sudsy water. Don't leave dirty dishes in the sink overnight.

- Pick up your pet's food dish promptly and wash it in hot sudsy water.

- Keep garbage and trash in containers with tight-fitting lids. Dispose of garbage and recyclables regularly.

- Don't let newspapers, magazines, paper grocery bags, boxes, or other items pile up to provide hiding and breeding areas for cockroaches.

For additional excellent information on cockroach management, see the Resource Guide.

INDOOR MOLDS

Molds, along with mushrooms and yeast, are microscopic fungi that are present everywhere, indoors and outdoors. Molds need a food source to grow (any organic material will do) and they gradually destroy whatever they grow on. Mold spores are common inside homes. They will grow and multiply when sufficient moisture and organic material is present. Indoor mold sources include leaky plumbing, damp basements or bathrooms, damp clothes in a hamper, refrigerator trays, beneath water-damaged surfaces, behind walls, floors, ceilings, upholstered furniture, damp closets, carpets (especially the backing or padding), air conditioners and humidifiers—the list is endless.

If you see discolored patches or speckled growth on walls or furniture, or if you smell a musty odor, take steps to eliminate moisture and to clean and remove the mold. Protect yourself by wearing rubber gloves and a mask with a HEPA filter to avoid inhaling airborne spores. Discard extremely moldy items. Scrub all others with soap or detergent in hot water, and disinfect with a solution of 1 cup of household bleach per gallon of water. Keep the disinfectant on for about 10 minutes to kill the mold spores, then rinse and dry thoroughly. Air out your house during and after the work, and take a fresh-air break often. HEPA filters are very efficient in trapping mold spores and dehumidifiers decrease humidity in damp areas.

SEASONAL ALLERGIC RHINITIS

Seasonal allergic rhinitis is caused by sensitivity to pollens, trees, grasses, and weeds, or to airborne mold spores. Seasonal allergic rhinitis is more commonly called hay fever, but despite the name, symptoms are not caused by hay and are not usually accompanied by fever. Ragweed is the main culprit, affecting 75 percent of seasonal allergic rhinitis sufferers. North America is host to numerous ragweed species which are found in most states. Each plant produces about a million pollen grains during an average season. Symptoms generally crop up in spring, summer, and early autumn although allergy seasons vary depending on where you live as well as the type of plants and trees in your area. In southern states, it can begin as early as January. When pollen sensitive individuals are repeatedly exposed to pollens, symptoms occur more frequently as the season progresses. This is called the "priming effect," because it takes fewer and fewer quantities of pollen to trigger a reaction. For instance, at the beginning of pollen season, it may take several hundred grains of pollen in the air to trigger a reaction, but at the end of the season it may take just a few. And once primed, you're more likely to react to lower exposure levels of other allergens, including those from your pet and dust mites.

OUTDOOR MOLDS

Outdoor molds are microscopic members of plants called *fungi*. They grow on cut grass, rotting or decaying leaves or vegetation, compost piles, hay bales, and in extremely shady areas. They release countless lightweight spores that travel through the air; some attach themselves to certain weeds and grasses. Although mold allergies tend to be worse in the fall after ragweed has cleared from the air, when it is damp and dead leaves provide a source of food, there is no "mold season" as there is a ragweed season. Mold is present on a year-round basis in the southern and western United States.

How to Avoid Airborne Pollens and Molds

- During pollen season, try to stay indoors with windows closed as much as possible between 5 and 10 A.M. Pollen counts tend to be highest early in the morning.

- Don't use fans in your home during pollen season; these draw in pollens and molds.

- Avoid parks with lots of trees and grass, and damp woods and shores. Minimize outdoor activities like jogging, hiking, or other strenuous exercise when the pollen count is high or on windy days when dust and pollens are circulating in the air. If you must be outdoors in these areas, wear a protective mask with a HEPA filter to help purify the air and keep pollen and mold spores out of your nose and mouth.

- Mowing grass, raking leaves, and gardening stir up pollens and mold. If you do these activities, wear a long-sleeved shirt, long pants, gloves, a mask with a HEPA filter, and sunglasses or, better yet, have a nonallergic family member do them.

- Pollen adheres to everything—your clothes, shoes, skin, and hair. Clothes are pollen magnets; change as soon as you come indoors. Shower and shampoo to cleanse off pollens that may be clinging to your skin and hair.

- Don't keep too many indoor plants, especially African violets, as molds grow on the damp soil, dead leaves, and the surface of clay pots.

Some allergy sufferers may experience both perennial and seasonal allergic rhinitis, in which case the perennial symptoms tend to worsen during specific pollen seasons. For example, you might have an allergy to your cat or dog that doesn't bother you most of the year but, during pollen season when you're sneezing repeatedly and your nose is runny or stuffy, even a brief encounter with your pet can cause symptoms.

TWELVE

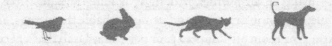

ALLERGEN-PROOFING YOUR HOME
A Room-by-Room Guide

Minimizing allergens on your pet and around the pet's environment, as you learned in previous chapters, is the first important step you can take to manage your symptoms. Allergy control doesn't stop there, however, because people are rarely allergic only to animals. The next course of action is to reduce your exposure to other allergens in your home. The more of them you can remove—*especially dust, dust mite, mold, and pollen allergens*—the better. You may not be able to completely eliminate all the other substances that aggravate your sensitivities, but with a little effort, you can minimize your exposure to them. It's not hard to do. Innovative built-in features such as vacuum bags that capture small allergens, cleaning fluid dispensers, electrostatic dusting cloths, and more make it easier to cut allergen buildup as well as cleaning time. It's no longer necessary to "mop till you drop."

Here is some general advice for allergy-proofing your house, followed by specific room-by-room tips. Ideally, have someone else do all the necessary cleaning. If that's not possible, wear a dust mask that covers your nose and mouth to avoid inhaling heavy doses of allergens. Don't be intimidated by the many suggestions. Unless your allergies are severe, *you'll probably need to observe only a few.* Just turning your bedroom into an allergy-free zone—using an air purifier, making it as mite- and dust-free as possible, removing carpeting and using washable throw rugs, and declaring the room off-limits to your pet—may be all that's necessary to live more comfortably with the pet you love without changing your pattern of living and without the need for medication. Most of the special products mentioned in this chapter are available from the mail-order allergy supply catalogs listed in the Resource Guide.

GENERAL GUIDELINES

HEPA Purifiers

Because pet allergens—*especially Fel d 1*—lightly float through the indoor air, invisible to the naked eye, a HEPA cleaner can be a tremendous help in purifying the air. High Efficiency Particulate Air purifiers have the capacity to filter out submicron particles. A "true" HEPA filter can capture particles 0.3 microns in size with 99.97 percent efficiency. Anything less is *not* a true HEPA and must be referred to as "HEPA-type." Place a HEPA purifier in your bedroom as well as in other rooms where your pet spends time.

Dust and Dusting

Dust is a mixture of many substances in a home environment. One speck of ordinary house dust that you see in a shaft of sunlight may contain bacteria, feathers, dust mite waste, insect particles, pollen, skin scales, hair, animal dander, lint, dried food particles, in short whatever happens to be floating in the air—any or all of which may be allergenic. Use damp cloths or electrostatic cleaning cloths and mops that retain dust without stirring it up. Dust thoroughly at least once a week: on top and under the furniture, window frames and sills, hard floors and baseboards, the tops of doors and lamp shades.

Vacuum Cleaners

Most conventional vacuum cleaners rate below par when it comes to retaining the microscopic particles, found by the millions in carpets, which trigger allergic reactions. Their filtering systems are only capable of retaining particles of 50 microns or larger, when much smaller particles—*Fel d 1 cat allergen in particular*—are the ones that aggravate you the most. Conventional vacuums do pick up small irritants, but they blow them through the exhaust outlet right back into the air, aggravating the allergies you're trying to relieve. You can, however, turn a standard vacuum into an allergy fighter by switching to double-lined, high-efficiency vacuum bags that augment filtration. These are available for most upright and canister models. If your allergies are serious, your best choice for removing dirt and pet allergens is an "allergy vacuum," with built-in, sealed true HEPA filtration system. Allergy sufferers should avoid personally changing vacuum bags, and should stay out of a room for thirty minutes after it is vacuumed.

Carpets, Floors, and Walls

Carpets are major allergen reservoirs. They hold 100 times more allergens than nonporous flooring. Small particles of Fel d 1, dander, dust, dust mite skeletons or excreta, mold, and pollen pile up deep inside the fibers (often to the padding underneath) and become very difficult to remove. The best choices are carpets with low pile, or short shags, or throw rugs that can be washed or shaken outdoors regularly.

Consider replacing carpets, especially in your bedroom, with laminate, vinyl, tile, wood, or other hard flooring that can be damp mopped at least twice a week. If removing carpeting isn't an option, vacuum every other day. Work against the pile, stroking several times over each area, overlapping movements to capture as many allergens as possible. Use the crevice attachment in corners.

An easy way to control pet odors and leave carpets smelling fresh is to sprinkle a deodorizing product such as Arm & Hammer Pet Fresh Carpet & Room Deodorizer evenly over your carpet, wait 15 minutes, then vacuum thoroughly. A number of other treatments and cleaners are available that neutralize animal dander, dust mite, pollen, and mold allergens in carpets and render them harmless to you, your pets, and your environment. Room-sized and wall-to-wall carpeting should be professionally dry-cleaned or steam-cleaned every year.

Furnishings and Curtains

Minimize overstuffed sofas and chairs, furniture upholstered with rough-textured fabrics, and other ornate furnishings. Use washable curtains made of cotton or synthetic fabrics that can be taken down and laundered frequently to eliminate dust and dust mites. Avoid long or heavy drapes and venetian or other kinds of vertical slatted blinds that attract dust and allergens. Use washable roller blinds instead. If you do have drapes, open the folds and vacuum each panel with the brush attachment. Pay special attention to the part of the drapes and the hem where dust and loose pet hair can accumulate. Reduce allergens dust in curtains and drapes by tumbling them in a cool dryer for a few minutes.

Walls

Choose painted walls over wallpaper, and wipe them down regularly with a damp sponge or vacuum them with the hand tool attachments, especially if you own a cat. Fel d 1 is a sticky allergen that adheres to walls once it settles.

Air Vents

Cover air vents and furnace registers tightly with cheesecloth, nylon, or other thin material to create a filter to capture pet allergens and dust and keep them from circulating through your air-conditioning or heating systems. You can also buy vent guards and electrostatic filters to prevent allergens from circulating. The latter can be cut to fit the size of the air vents in any room.

Dehumidifiers

If your allergies are severe, a dehumidifier can be a big help in reducing the mite population inside your home, especially in the bedroom. Dust mites need lots of indoor moisture to live and multiply. Lower the indoor humidity to 50 percent or less and they're in trouble. Mold and mildew is also controlled since both need high humidity levels to thrive. Lower humidity reduces mildew odor as well. Clean the unit frequently to prevent mold growth.

Other Irritants

Avoid being exposed to other irritants such as perfumes, air fresheners, tobacco smoke, pesticides and other aerosol sprays, chemicals, and paint fumes, as these can trigger allergy symptoms. Cigarette smoke itself is an allergen. If you smoke, quit! Plants can contain mold spores and pollen. Don't allow dead leaves to remain in potted plants. Mold growth can also occur within the soil and from overwatering. Covering the surface of the soil with decorative stones or bark chips will prevent mold spores from floating into the air as well as discourage pets from using potted plants as litter boxes.

And now, some advice for specific rooms. . . .

THE BEDROOM

The first and most important room to allergen-proof is the bedroom, because you spend about a third of your time there. It's also the room that contains the greatest number of dust mites and pet allergens, especially if you have allowed your dog or cat to sleep on the bed in the past. The Mayo Clinic estimates that one double bed alone may contain up to 2 million dust mites! And large numbers of dust mites are also found in sheets, pillowcases, and blankets.

- Encase mattresses, box springs, and pillows in airtight, zippered mite-proof covers. Even if you have a bedroom dehumidifier, your body moisture and skin scales provide the necessary humidity and food for mites to thrive inside your mattress and pillow. Dust mite allergens can escape through the zippers; many doctors recommend taping the edges of the encasings. If the mattress is not covered, vacuum it once a week. Use the vacuum's wand or upholstery attachment and pay special attention to indented or buttoned areas where dust collects.

- Use only washable bed linens: sheets, pillowcases, blankets, comforters, and mattress pads. Change weekly and wash them in hot water (140°F) alone or use ¾ ounce of De-Mite laundry additive in hot, warm, or cold water to wash out mites and their allergenic waste. Tumble dry in a hot or warm dryer.

- Wipe all parts of the bed thoroughly with a damp cloth or an electrostatic dust cloth to prevent dust buildup.

- Do not store anything under your bed.

- Keep furniture to a minimum; the more washable surfaces the better.

- The fewer objects displayed the better: keep dressers and nightstands free of books, magazines and other papers, knickknacks, jewelry boxes, collectibles, dried flowers and potted plants, and beds free of decorative pillows. *These are all dust magnets*. Store them in drawers or closed cabinets.

- If the allergic person is a child, avoid stuffed toys that accumulate dust. Use washable toys and store them in a closed toy chest. Stuffed animals that a child can't bear to part with should be tumbled in a warm dryer on a weekly basis.

- Air out the room on a regular basis, except on days when the pollen count is high.

- Dust regularly under the bed, behind dressers, chests, nightstands, baseboards. Don't forget ceiling fans, as dust and allergens collect on the tops.

- The dust mite population in a bedroom carpet is much higher than in other rooms. If you can only remove carpeting in one room, let it be the bedroom. Replace with washable area rugs or hard flooring. Otherwise, vacuum at least once a week.

BEDROOM CLOSETS

- Keep bedroom closets as dust-free as the bedroom.
- Downsize. It's normal to have amassed a quantity of clothing, books, and other items over the years. Start by emptying everything out of your closet. Divide it into three parts: things to keep, things to donate to charity or send to consignment, and items to throw out.
- Hang only *washable* clothing of the current season in the closet. Keep dry-cleaned clothing in zippered plastic garment bags. Store out-of-season clothing and furs elsewhere.
- Do not use mothballs or moth crystals.
- Store shoes in boxes, on racks, or in hanging bags off the floor.
- Check floors, shelves, and boxes for mold or mildew.
- Don't store luggage, cleaning appliances, or chemicals in the bedroom closet.
- Keep the closet door shut.

These same principles apply to all closets in your home.

THE LIVING ROOM/FAMILY ROOM

The living room and family room are other important areas in which your pets—dogs and cats especially—frequently curl up beside you on the couch or in your favorite chair while you read, watch TV, play video games, or just doze off for a nap.

- Try not to let pets sleep on the couch or chairs. When you close your bedroom door at night to keep out your dog or cat, you may not know where your pet goes to rest or sleep. Consider encasing the couch or upholstered armchairs with plastic or washable coverings to keep allergens from accumulating.

- Keep furniture to a minimum. Simple designs attract less dust.

- Reduce the number of dust traps, like rough-textured fabrics, piles of newspapers, books, or magazines, decorative pillows, heavy drapes or curtains, knickknacks, and potted plants.

- Follow the advice in chapter 4 about vacuuming, dusting, carpets, floors, walls, and curtains.

- Take proper care of fireplaces and chimneys. Corrosion inside them can slow down the flow of exhaust gases and allow dangerous fumes to flow back inside. Gas fireplaces should be vented properly to prevent any soot or carbon monoxide from leaking into the home. Also, wood smoke can irritate allergy and asthma sufferers. Hardwoods release the fewest emissions; pine wood produces the most and can create a creosote buildup. Store wood outdoors—split, stacked, and protected from the rain—to keep it from becoming moldy or contaminated with insects.

THE BATHROOM

The most serious problems in the bathroom are moisture and the development of mold.

- Keep bathroom door open when not in use to improve air circulation.

- Shower stalls and shower curtains are notorious for being breeding grounds for mold and mildew. After use, squeegee or sponge shower walls dry. If your shower curtain or liner is mildewed, replace it. Prevent mold growth on new curtains or liners by soaking them in salt water before hanging. Better yet, use a heavy-duty curtain that inhibits the growth of mold, mildew, and bacteria.

- A dehumidifier will help to remove excess humidity produced by bathing or showering; otherwise keep the bathroom window open while you are showering.

- Clean the tub, toilet, shower stall, tile, walls, floor, window frames and sills, and any other surfaces weekly with a disinfectant cleaner formulated to kill mold and mildew. Consider using No More Mildew, a nontoxic, micro-thin sealant spray that works on any surface where mold grows for up to two full years.

- Check under the bathroom cabinet and around and behind the toilet to be sure there are no leaks or mold growth. Repair all leaks.

- Add an extra towel rack to spread wet towels so they dry more quickly. Hang up the bath mat to dry, too, after bathing or showering; standing on it while you're wet can lead to mold growth.

THE KITCHEN

The kitchen is a prime area for the development of mold due to moisture as well as food. Another problem in the kitchen is cockroaches (see chapter 11, "Other Substances That Make Pet Allergies Worse").

- Leave an open box of baking soda in the refrigerator for deodorizing. Replace it every three months.

- Mold can grow in the refrigerator, especially around the doors. Use an all-purpose cleaner or a solution of ½ cup of household bleach mixed with a gallon of water to clean the door gasket (the rubber bumper that seals the door shut). Use the same solution to clean the walls and shelves. Empty drip trays frequently; adding salt will help prevent mold growth. Two or three times a year, vacuum the condenser coils (at the back) to remove dust and pet hair buildup.

- Clean the dishwasher and other appliances regularly with the bleach solution.

- Use an exhaust fan over the stove (vented to the outside) or open a window to remove excess steam and odors when cooking.

- Empty and clean garbage pails frequently. Sprinkle borax powder in the bottom.

- Damp kitchen towels, dishcloths, and sponges are magnets for allergens and bacteria. Change towels/dishcloths often; launder them in hot water and detergent. Clean sponges with bleach or in the dishwasher, or zap them for a few seconds in the microwave.

LAUNDRY ROOM, BASEMENT, AND GARAGE

Like the bathroom, a damp laundry room, basement, or garage provides the ideal conditions for the growth of mold and bacteria.

- Use detergents that are free of perfumes and dyes.
- Avoid using fabric softeners because of their strong scents.
- Vent your clothes dryer to the outdoors to avoid dispersing lint in the house.
- Dry clothes in the clothes dryer, not outside, as doing so may attract pollens, molds, and other airborne pollutants.
- Don't let damp clothing pile up and don't store anything damp in your laundry hamper, otherwise it quickly becomes a source of mold growth.
- Keep the laundry room, basement, and garage as uncluttered as possible. Throw out all unnecessary items. Store out-of-season clothing in vinyl storage bags and other items on shelves away from the walls and floor. Newspapers, boxes, and other things stored on a concrete floor can become moldy from condensation.

- Inspect pipes and repair any leaks.
- Have furnace ducts, air-conditioning units, and electrostatic filters serviced and cleaned regularly.
- Add a HEPA filter to your heating unit and change it frequently.
- Avoid exposure to vehicle exhaust. Always keep the door from the garage to the house closed tight.

THIRTEEN

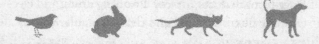

PET ALLERGIES IN THE WORKPLACE

Next to the bedroom, adult allergy sufferers probably spend the most time in their workplaces. It would be perfect if they could avoid professions that regularly expose them to allergens, but that is not always the case. Sensitivities to animals can present an issue for obvious occupations such as veterinarians and veterinary technicians; professional dog and cat groomers; jockeys, horse grooms, and stable workers; animal and poultry breeders; farmers; livestock workers; zoo and circus workers; laboratory technicians; research scientists and other animal-facility workers, who are all at risk of being exposed to high levels of potent animal allergens on a regular basis. Less obvious potential workplace difficulties are often found in schools, pediatric hospitals, and nursing and retirement homes that keep pets such as hamsters, mice, or gerbils which may cause them to be loaded with pet allergens.

Allergies in the workplace can cause problems for both employees and employers by impacting production. Various studies have shown, for instance, that 11 to 30 percent of individuals regularly exposed to laboratory animals experience symptoms. Rats and mice are the most allergenic and the primary cause of these problems. Urinary proteins produced by rodents are especially potent allergens; tests have shown that they are present in large quantities that become airborne quickly. Rabbits and guinea pigs also shed dander and deposit saliva on their fur through licking.

A high percentage of jockeys, grooms, and stable workers develop allergies and asthma. Their sensitivities are triggered not only by the dander and urine of horses, but also by mold spores in damp hay as well as allergens in the grasses and grains that horses eat. If mice or other rodents are present in stables or barns, their urine may cause additional adverse reactions.

The best way to reduce animal allergen levels in the workplace is to contain the source of production. The sooner you can avoid or reduce your exposure to animal dander, salivary, and urinary secretions at work, the better you can control your allergies or asthma. Here are some suggestions from the National Institute for Occupational Safety and Health (NIOSH) that can help reduce exposure:

- Reduce skin contact by wearing protective clothing: lab coats, gloves, and approved particulate respirators with face shields.

- Do not wear street clothes at work, especially if you handle animals.

- Leave work clothes at your workplace.

- Keep cages and animal areas clean. Wear masks, especially when cleaning cages.

- Use absorbent pads for bedding or corncob bedding instead of sawdust or straw.

- Try to work with an animal species or sex that is known to be less allergenic than others.

- Ventilate animal cages and handling areas separately from the rest of the facility. Direct airflow toward the

backs of the cages and away from workers. Install
ventilated cage racks or filter-top animal cages.

- Shower after work and wash your hair.

More technical information about preventing allergy and
asthma in pet handlers can be accessed on the NIOSH website:
www.cdc.gov/niosh/animalrt.html.

Minor problems in air ventilation can cause major health problems. You may be inhaling pet allergens because the heating or air-
conditioning is not working properly. In most buildings with
central heating, ventilation, and air-conditioning (HVAC) systems, the quality of air circulation depends entirely on the opera-
tion and maintenance of this equipment. If windows cannot be
opened, faulty HVAC systems can spray large quantities of pet allergen particles into the environment. Keeping a small HEPA filter
in your immediate work area can also improve air quality. Pet allergens often attach to small particles that tend to remain suspended
in the air, making them available to trap in the filter. Even aside
from pet allergen concerns, research on modern airtight buildings
suggests that between building materials, air-purifying systems,
faulty ventilation, office furnishings, and certain machines, indoor
air is often polluted with allergens. Bearing in mind that allergies
are cumulative, when you count the number of irritants you are exposed to day after day, they often add up to enormous doses,
enough for any allergy sufferer to exceed his or her tolerance level
and to trigger attacks.

Allergic workers should try to modify the tasks they perform:
for example, cleaning cages and handling animals while they're
sleeping exposes workers to fifty to one hundred times fewer allergens than when the animals are active. Stable workers who handle
baled hay (contaminated by dust, pollens, and mold spores)

should wear protective masks and gloves, and wash their hands, arms, and clothing afterward. Horse droppings should be regularly picked up. The stable itself should have a free flow of air from front to back and side to side.

The reasonable use of preventative medications may also help to control symptoms. Individuals with mild sensitivities who can predetermine their exposure to animals may be able to medicate themselves with over-the-counter preparations before arriving at their workplace. An allergist can prescribe medications to control more serious allergy and asthma symptoms at work and, in addition, can advise about avoiding or at least reducing exposure to workplace allergens.

FOURTEEN

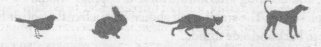

WHEN TO SEE A DOCTOR

Allergies to pets and other airborne substances can often be relieved by making certain environmental adjustments, but the time may come when your sensitivities are severe enough to require the attention of a physician. You should consult a doctor when your symptoms become frequent and irritating enough to hamper your daily activities.

Many allergies are handled first by primary care physicians or pediatricians who are most familiar with a patient's medical history. When symptoms persist or increase in magnitude, however, your doctor may refer you to a board-certified allergist, a physician with advanced training in allergy and immunology.

Until recently, it's been an almost automatic response for many allergists to instruct patients to immediately "get rid" of their pets. This attitude has changed considerably in recent years, not only because of the new developments that have taken place in the field of allergy and immunology, but also the increasing awareness of the importance of pets to the emotional and physical well-being of people.

Today, many allergists are much more sensitive to the relationships between patients and their companion animals. When communicating with your allergist, let him or her know your goals in treating and controlling your symptoms. If your symptoms are not severe or debilitating, it is not unreasonable to explain to your specialist that your goal is to minimize bothersome symptoms while keeping your pet. If a physician's only or primary suggestion is to remove your pet from your home, then you may wish to obtain a second opinion from another specialist who is willing to work with you on intermediary steps first.

WHAT TO EXPECT AT THE PHYSICIAN'S OFFICE

A thorough and accurate medical diagnosis is of the utmost importance when you have allergies. This not only helps your physician determine the best course of prevention and treatment, but also helps you to understand your specific allergy triggers and how to manage them. Generally speaking, the diagnostic procedure begins with the physician taking a detailed medical, family, and environmental history, followed by a pertinent physical examination and concluding with one or more skin tests or blood tests. To help control your allergies, it's critical to identify all the allergens responsible for provoking your symptoms, so your doctor can design a treatment program specifically for you.

ALLERGY TESTS

Your allergist may use one or more tests to pinpoint the specific substances you are allergic to. Some of the most important tests for diagnosing allergies to pets and other airborne substances are discussed in this section.

Prick or Puncture and Intradermal Skin Tests

Skin tests are the oldest, fastest, and most widely accepted method of allergy testing. The test takes about 5 minutes to apply and is read 15 minutes after application. Several days prior to the skin testing, patients are asked to temporarily discontinue taking certain medications—particularly antihistamines—as the presence of these drugs in the body can interfere with results. A list of other medications to withhold is usually provided by the medical practice. Be sure to provide your allergist with a complete list of all of your current medications, including over-the-counter preparations, prior to skin testing.

Before beginning, the test sites of the skin—usually the inside of the forearm or upper part of the back—are wiped with alcohol (to remove skin oils that can make ink and allergen material run off), allowed to dry by evaporation, and then marked with a pen in vertical rows to indicate where each allergen will be applied.

In the *prick* or *puncture test,* a diluted drop of each allergen being tested (for example, Fel d 1, animal dander, dust mites, pollens, or molds) is placed next to the marked areas on the skin. A drop of a saline (saltwater) solution is also applied as a "negative control" and histamine as a "positive control," against which the potential allergen sites are read. A nurse or technician uses a small plastic pricking device to penetrate the surface of the skin, just enough so the allergen solution can enter and interact with the skin, but not so deep as to cause bleeding. If you're being tested for multiple substances, separate devices are used for each test to avoid mixing of allergens.

If the test is negative, the area on the skin remains flat and with minimal to little redness. If the test is positive, sensitized tissue mast cells will react with the allergen-causing histamine and other allergy-provoking mediators which produce the classic "wheal-and-flare" reaction on the skin (a raised itchy bump, or *wheal*, surrounded by a reddened area, or *flare*) within 15 minutes. Generally, the larger the reaction, the more sensitive you are. Reactions are always measured against those of the control sites. Suppose you are being tested for cats and mold, for instance. If you are allergic to cats but not to mold, the puncture where the cat allergen penetrated your skin will itch and produce a mosquito-bite type of reaction, while the puncture with mold allergen, as well as the control site, will not show significant site bumps and redness compared to the controls.

Intradermal skin testing is sometimes performed when suspected allergens do not produce significant positive reactions with a prick or puncture test. The skin test sites are wiped with alcohol, and more diluted solutions of the allergens are injected with a fine needle just below the surface of the skin into the forearm or the side of the upper arm. If the reaction is positive, the skin reddens and swells slightly to form welts, in the wheal-and-flare reaction previously described. Results are apparent within 15 to 20 minutes, after which time the size of the wheals and amount of skin redness are measured.

Skin tests usually produce swelling and itching around the puncture site; if significant discomfort develops, a spray with lidocaine can be applied to stop the itching. A mild cortisone cream can be applied later at home if the area continues to itch. A systemic reaction rarely develops, but if it does, your allergist can provide immediate assistance.

RAST Test

Your allergist may also choose a blood test to help diagnose your allergies. This test is called a *RAST* (radioallergosorbent) test, which measures the levels of specific IgE (allergy-provoked anti-body) produced in response to allergens to which you may be sensitive. Very simply put, if this test detects elevated levels of IgE antibodies in the blood, an allergy is likely. Blood tests are utilized when skin rashes (extensive hives or eczema) preclude skin testing, when allergy symptoms are so severe that the patient cannot discontinue taking antihistamines, or when the risk of a systemic reaction (a severe allergic reaction called *anaphylaxis*) makes skin testing dangerous.

RAST tests have several disadvantages: they are more expensive than skin tests, they take longer to obtain results (two to three days), they can be less sensitive than skin tests, and they produce more false-positive results.

Results and Treatment

Your doctor will interpret the results of your tests in light of your allergy history and physical exam findings, and advise you how to manage your allergy symptoms. Doctors use several approaches to help allergy sufferers: (1) advise them how to minimize or avoid the allergen as much as possible, (2) prescribe medication to relieve symptoms, and (3) when these measures do not effectively control the symptoms, prescribe specific allergen immunotherapy or "allergy shots" to help achieve desensitization of one's allergies. There is no cure for allergies, but one or a combination of these approaches will usually provide relief.

FIFTEEN

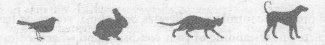

WHAT PROFESSIONALS ARE DOING TO ALLEVIATE ALLERGIES

If you are allergic to hairy, furry, or feathered animals, taking the steps to minimize allergens on your pet(s) and making a few changes in your home (steps previously outlined in this book) may be all that's necessary to control your allergies. If this strategy doesn't significantly reduce your symptoms, however, your allergist may recommend combining these measures with medications.

ALLERGY AND ASTHMA MEDICATIONS

This is a very promising time for the treatment of allergies and asthma, especially for sensitivities to pets and other airborne allergens. Recent studies have led to new ways of viewing these conditions and more effective medications to treat them. Dozens of new, effective prescription and over-the-counter drugs are now available to make living with allergies and animals much more comfortable.

Here is a brief description of some medications used to treat allergies and asthma. This information is intended to help you understand the most common types of medications your doctor may recommend. It is *not* a substitute for professional medical advice. Asthma, especially, is a serious illness that needs to be carefully monitored by a doctor.

Ask Questions and Learn the Facts

To properly control your allergies or asthma, you must have a complete understanding of your condition and what medication and strategies can best treat it. Your doctor should receive a list of *all* prescription drugs, over-the-counter preparations, and vitamin, mineral, or herbal supplements you are taking—anything that might affect your use of a newly prescribed medication.

Don't hesitate to ask questions. Find out the brand and generic name of each drug your doctor prescribes and learn as much about it as you can: what it is supposed to do, how and when you should take it, how long it takes to bring relief, how long the medication should be used, and if there are any warnings or precautions. Ask about any side effects and interactions with other medicines, food, or dietary supplements, and what can be done to avoid them. And never start or stop taking any medication without first speaking with your doctor.

Antihistamines

Antihistamines have been around for over fifty years and are the most commonly used drugs to provide symptomatic relief from allergies. They are available over-the-counter (OTC) and by prescription as tablets, liquids, chewables, nasal sprays, and eyedrops. Divided into sedating and non-sedating, antihistamines block the action of histamine and other chemicals released by your mast cells during an allergic reaction (see chapter 1, "Understanding Allergy and Asthma"), hence the name *anti,* or against, and *histamine.* They help to relieve or prevent the symptoms associated with allergic rhinitis—sneezing; itchy eyes, nose, and throat; and postnasal drip.

OTC antihistamines, unfortunately, can generate a number of unwanted side effects, including drowsiness, dry mouth, and constipation. Impaired motor coordination due to drowsiness can occur, thus it is paramount to heed label warnings not to drive a car while taking sedating antihistamines. The newer non-sedating antihistamines have become the largest class of these medications.

Nasal Decongestants

These medications are available both over-the-counter and by prescription in tablet, liquid, and nasal spray form. They work by constricting small blood vessels in the lining of the nasal and sinus passages, thereby reducing swelling and alleviating congestion to make breathing easier. However, because they alone do not block the release of histamines or other chemical mediators during an allergic reaction, decongestants are often combined with antihistamines in a single medication. Decongestants can cause anxiety, irritability, dry mouth, insomnia, heart racing, and an increase in blood pressure. The American Academy of Allergy Asthma & Immunology recommends that OTC decongestant nasal sprays not be used for more than three days in a row. They open a stuffy nose so quickly that many individuals become dependent and keep using them beyond the three-day time span. "Rebound rhinitis" can then occur as blood vessels in the nasal lining swell again, leading an individual to spray more and more often to open the nose, with declining and shorter-lived responses and worsening congestion.

Eyedrops

Allergies to pets frequently affect the conjunctiva (the red lining of the inside of the eyelids), causing itching, tearing, swelling, and redness. Cleansing your eyes with artificial tears (which contain no medicine) may temporarily flush away allergens and relieve symptoms, but you may need drops containing antihistamines or decongestants. Do not, however, use OTC eye-drops with decongestants beyond a three-day time span because, like nasal decongestants, long-term use can cause a rebound effect. If OTC preparations don't work, ask your doctor about prescription eyedrops. Several classes of medications are available for treatment; those containing antihistamines or mast cell stabilizers are very effective in reducing symptoms.

Mast Cell Stabilizers: Cromolyn Sodium and Nedocromil Sodium

These anti-inflammatory drugs work by stabilizing the mast cells and inhibiting the release of histamine and other chemicals upon exposure to certain triggers. *Cromolyn sodium* is available as over-the-counter nasal spray (NasalCrom), and eyedrops (Opticrom), and as a prescription dry-powder inhaler, and a liquid that is inhaled by nebulizer to treat asthma. It is FDA-approved for use in adults and children age five or older. *Nedocromil* (Tilade), available as an inhaler, is a similar drug that is FDA-approved for use in adults and children age twelve or older for the treatment of asthma.

Unlike antihistamines and decongestants, which relieve ongoing symptoms, cromolyn and nedocromil are preventive agents that must be taken for several weeks before reaching maximum effectiveness. If, for instance, your mother-in-law is allergic to your cat and her symptoms flare up each time she visits you, a few puffs of NasalCrom, a cromolyn nasal spray, into each nostril, starting several days before she enters your home, may offer protection. Neither drug should be used for the immediate relief of an allergy or asthma attack. What makes these medications so desirable is their remarkable safety record; they are well tolerated in most cases, rarely causing side effects.

Leukotriene Inhibitors

Leukotriene inhibitors are the newest class of treatment options, developed in the 1990s. These anti-inflammatory medications block the action of leukotrienes, potent chemicals released by the mast cells during an allergic reaction. According to the AAAAI, leukotrienes block both the early responses to allergic triggers (itching and sneezing) and the delayed response (congestion). Leukotriene inhibitors are prescribed as a long-term preventive agent and are used as a controlled medication for asthma as well as allergic rhinitis.

Corticosteroids

Corticosteroids, also called steroids, are highly effective anti-inflammatory medications for the treatment of allergies and asthma. They are prescribed for both short- and long-term use to reduce symptoms in patients with allergic rhinitis and chronic moderate to severe asthma. Steroids are available in topical creams and ointments (for skin allergies), eyedrops (for allergic conjunctivitis), nasal sprays (for allergic rhinitis), as well as tablets, liquid inhalers, and a nebulized solution (for asthma). It is important to know that the corticosteroids described here are *not* the same as the anabolic steroids used—perhaps "misused" is a better term—by some athletes to enhance their performance.

Steroid nasal sprays treat allergic and nonallergic rhinitis, and are effective in preventing symptoms of nasal congestion, runny nose, itching, and sneezing when taken on a regular basis. Packaged in easy-to-use pocket-sized pump spray bottles, they are the most effective nasal medications currently available. Several nasal steroids are FDA-approved for use in patients six years of age and older, with dosage amounts determined by the doctor.

Topical cream and lotion steroids, available OTC (milder) or by prescription, relieve the symptoms of rashes and other skin irritations, such as eczema or contact dermatitis.

Inhaled corticosteroids are asthma medications designed to be inhaled into the lungs as long-term controlled medication to treat and prevent inflammation of the airways. They provide symptom control and have far fewer side effects and long-term risks than oral steroids. Available only by prescription, inhaled steroids are administered via either a metered-dose inhaler (MDI), a hand-held pressurized pocket-sized canister that delivers medication via the mouth into the lungs, or a compressor-powered nebulizer that transforms liquid medication into a fine mist spray that is inhaled into the lungs. Using corticosteroid inhalers can produce minor side effects, which include cough, hoarseness, and thrush (a fungal infection that appears as creamy white patches in the mouth). These side effects can be reduced or prevented by gargling and rinsing your mouth with water after each use of the spray. A device called a "spacer" can also be attached to the mouthpiece of an inhaler to improve the delivery of the medication to your lungs and reduce these potential side effects.

Oral steroids, such as prednisone, generally cause more side effects than topical creams, sprays, and inhalers. They are usually prescribed for short-term use (a few days to weeks) when a patient's allergies or asthma is severe or out of control and other treatment measures have failed. They should not be used for prolonged periods of time unless absolutely necessary, as they can cause such serious side effects as weight gain, fluid retention, short stature in children, osteoporosis, hypertension, glaucoma, and hypo-adrenalism. Women are particularly susceptible to developing osteoporosis and related bone fractures, although any patient can be at risk. Extended therapy is reserved for those rare patients with severe uncontrollable asthma.

Bronchodilators

Bronchodilators are inhaled medications used to alleviate symptoms of asthma attacks. Available by inhaler, nebulizer, pills, or injection, they work by relaxing the smooth bronchial muscles to allow more air to flow in and out of the lungs. Short-acting bronchodilators provide fast relief during an acute asthma attack and last three to four hours, while long-acting ones can have immediate or delayed onset effect, and provide up to 12 hours of relief. Bronchodilators are also used 15 to 20 minutes prior to exercise to prevent exercise-induced asthma symptoms. Some bronchodilators are approved for use in higher level sports competition, and athletes with asthma typically use them before events and, if necessary, again during or after them.

Theophylline

Theophylline is a bronchodilator that works primarily by relaxing the smooth bronchial muscles to open up the air passages. Theophylline is available in the form of pills, slow- or sustained-release capsules, and by injection. Unlike the adrenergic bronchodilators previously described, theophylline is not as fast acting during an asthma attack, and is more commonly prescribed for maintenance therapy. Theophylline is related to caffeine and can produce such side effects as headache, nervousness, sleeplessness, and elevated heart rate. You should avoid drinking large quantities of caffeinated coffee, tea, or colas while taking theophylline, as these may exacerbate the stimulant effects of this drug.

Combination Therapy

Single medications may not always be effective and doctors sometimes prescribe a combination of drugs that can provide better symptom control. Some asthmatics, for instance, take both an oral medication, such as a leukotriene modifier, and an inhaled steroid as their daily maintenance treatment. These drugs act synergistically when combined; in other words, the total effect is greater than that of either drug taken alone.

IMMUNOTHERAPY OR "ALLERGY SHOTS"

When the reasonable use of medications does not prove satisfactory in controlling your symptoms or the side effects of the medications are troublesome, your allergist may recommend allergen immunotherapy, commonly called "allergy shots," a proven and effective method to increase your tolerance to the substances that provoke your allergies.

The Goal of Immunotherapy

For pet owners, the goal of immunotherapy is to help you become desensitized to the specific animal allergens that cause your sensitivities and to tolerate your pet's presence with minimal, if any, discomfort. Immunotherapy does not cure allergies, but it can greatly reduce your sensitivities. It works like a vaccine. Your body reacts to injected amounts of the specific allergen, administered in gradually increasing doses, by developing a tolerance or immunity to that allergen. Once the tolerance level is reached, maintenance injections help keep symptoms in check, so that when you encounter your pet's allergens in the future, you'll experience a reduced response.

Which Allergies Respond Best

In general, people who suffer from allergic rhinitis are among the best candidates for immunotherapy; it is most effective for allergies to cats, dogs, dust mites, cockroaches, and a variety of pollens. And new allergens for pet desensitization are being developed that offer even greater success.

NEW CHEMICAL COMPOUND MAY END MISERY-MAKING CAT ALLERGIES

Dr. Andrew Saxon, chief of Clinical Immunology, and colleagues at the UCLA School of Medicine in Los Angeles have developed a breakthrough procedure for treating cat allergies.

The new treatment, reported in the April 2005 issue of *Nature Medicine*, involves linking Fel d 1 (cat allergen) to a human protein that effectively stops immune cells from releasing histamine, the chemical that provokes allergy symptoms. The compound, named GFD for *gamma Felis domesticus*, was tested in two types of mice specially bred to be allergic to cats and virtually blocked the histamine reaction that causes cat allergy symptoms in both types. According to Dr. Christopher Kepley, a coauthor of the report, a single injection blunted the allergic response before it began. Experiments with human cell cultures suggest it will do the same for people.

"This novel approach to treating cat allergies is encouraging news for millions of cat-allergic Americans," said Dr. Anthony Fauci, director of the National Institute of Allergy and Infectious Diseases, which funded the study. Cat allergy sufferers should hold off contacting their allergists, though. The treatment will not be available for at least three years.

How Often Shots Are Given

Immunotherapy requires an accurate diagnosis of your specific allergy, based on your medical and environmental history as well as skin test results. Once your allergist determines precisely which environmental allergens you are allergic to, he or she will prepare special mixtures that contain diluted extracts of the(se) specific allergen(s). The extracts—made from substances you are allergic to, such as Fel d 1, dog allergen, dust, or pollens—will then be injected via a small needle into your upper arm. The series of shots begins with small doses and gradually increases weekly until a maintenance level is reached. This is called the "buildup" phase, during which shots are usually given once or twice a week. The length of this phase generally ranges from three to six months.

Once the strongest dose, or maintenance level, is reached, shots are gradually reduced to every other week for one year, then every three weeks for one year, and then once monthly for one year. Your allergist will determine which schedule is best suited for you. Redness and swelling around the injection site is normal and should subside within 4 to 8 hours. Serious side effects rarely occur but, because the shots are made from extracts of the substance to which you are allergic, you will be asked to wait in your allergist's office for about 30 minutes following your shots to be sure there is no systemic reaction.

How Long Treatment Lasts

Immunotherapy requires a time commitment on the part of patients. The success of a regimen depends on a patient's receiving shots at regularly scheduled intervals. Most patients begin to experience significant relief within six months to one year after starting immunotherapy. Some patients experience symptom relief sooner. Talk to your allergist for more information.

Although immunotherapy alone can significantly reduce your allergy symptoms, it is even *more* effective if exposure to the offending allergens is also reduced. Continuing to practice the measures outlined in this book for minimizing allergens both on your pet and in your home will noticeably increase the effectiveness of your treatment.

RESOURCE GUIDE

As this book focuses on allergies to pets, you will want to learn more practical and medical information about the triggers, symptoms, treatment, and management of other allergies and asthma to lead an active and healthy life. Here are some of the best up-to-date print and online resources to check out. Internet references, addresses, and telephone numbers given in this section were accurate at the time the book went to press.

BOOKS

Ansorge, Rick, Eric Metcalf, and the Editors of Prevention Health Books. *Allergy Free Naturally*. Emmaus, PA: Rodale Inc., 2001.

Berger, William E., M.D. *Allergies and Asthma for Dummies*. Hoboken, NJ: Wiley Publishing Company, 2004.

Berger, William E., M.D., and Debra L. Gordon. *Allergy & Asthma Relief*. Pleasantville, NY: Reader's Digest Association, 2004.

Gamlin, Linda. *The Allergy Bible*. Pleasantville, NY: Reader's Digest Association, 2001.

Kalstone, Shirlee. *Good Cat! A Proven Guide to Successful Litter Box Use and Problem Solving*. Hoboken, NJ: Howell Book House, 2005.

Kalstone, Shirlee. *How to Housebreak Your Dog in 7 Days.* New York: Bantam Books, 2004.

May, Jeffrey C. *My House Is Killing Me.* Baltimore and London: The Johns Hopkins University Press, 2001.

Montague, Sara, and P. J. Dempsey. *The Complete Idiot's Guide to Horses.* Indianapolis, IN: Alpha Books, 2003.

Shepherd, Gillian, M.D., and Marian Betancourt. *What's in the Air?* New York: Pocket Books, 2002.

ALLERGY ORGANIZATIONS AND WEBSITES

Allergy & Asthma Network Mothers of Asthmatics: www.aanma.org

American Academy of Allergy Asthma & Immunology: www.aaaai.org

American College of Allergy, Asthma & Immunology: www.acaai.org

American Lung Association: www.lungusa.org

Asthma and Allergy Foundation of America: www.aafa.org

Centers for Disease Control and Prevention: www.cdc.gov

Environmental Protection Agency: www.epa.gov/iaq/molds/moldguide.html

National Institute of Allergy and Infectious Diseases: www.niaid.nih.gov

University of California Agricultural and Natural Resources Department: www.ipm.ucdavis.edu/index.html

WEBSITES

www.allergies.about.com/od/cats (More information on coping with cat allergies)

www.allergies.about.com/od/dogs (More information on coping with dog allergies) www.allerpet.com (Information, questions/answers, and more about allergies to all pets)

www.cavyspirit.com/allergies.htm (Information about living with Guinea Pig allergies)

www.equisearch.com/care/grooming (Caring for and grooming horses and more)

www.ferretcentral.org (Information on ferret care and allergies)

www.horse-sense.org (Newsletter on all phases of horse care)

www.hsus.org (The Humane Society of the United States)

www.ipm.ucdavis.edu/PMG/PESTNOTES/pn7467.html (Information on dealing with cockroaches)

www.petplace.com (Extensive information on all phases of caring for pets)

www.rabbit.org (Advice from the House Rabbit Society)

www.vetmedicine.about.com (Numerous articles on pet care)

ALLERGY PRODUCTS

Here are some major suppliers that stock a full line of allergy-related products. They are excellent sources for anti-dust mite protective encasings for pillows, mattresses, box springs; sheets and other bedding; items to control dust mites and animal allergens; mold and mildew inhibitors; dust and pollen masks; chemical-free cleaning products; air filters; allergy vacuums; and many other items.

Allergy Asthma Technology
8224 Lehigh Avenue
Morton Grove, IL 60053
Phone: 800-621-5545
www.allergyasthmatech.com

Allergy Control Products
96 Danbury Road
Ridgefield, CT 06877
Phone: 800-422-3878
www.allergycontrol.com

Allergy Relief Stores
Independence Mall
4201 Veterans Blvd., Suite A
Metairie, LA 70006
Phone: 800-555-0755
www.onlineallergyrelief.com

National Allergy Supply
1620-D Satellite Blvd.
Duluth, GA 30097
Phone: 800-522-1448
www.nationalallergy.com

PET PRODUCTS

In addition to PetSmart (www.petsmart.com) and Petco
(www.petco.com), here are three mail-order catalogs that stock almost everything for pets and will send you an illustrated catalog
on request. All accept major credit cards.

Brisky Pet Products
P.O. Box 186
Franklinville, NY 14737
Phone: 800-462-2464
www.brisky.com

Care-A-Lot Pet Supply Warehouse
1617 Diamond Springs Road
Virginia Beach, VA 23455
Phone: 800-343-7680
www.carealotpets.com

Drs. Foster & Smith
2253 Air Park Road, P.O. Box 100
Rhinelander, WI 54501-0100
Phone: 800-381-7179
www.drsfostersmith.com

J-B Wholesale Pet Supply
5 Raritan Road
Oakland, NJ 07436
Phone: 800-526-0388
www.jbpet.com

PetEdge
P.O. Box 128
Topsfield, MA 01983-0228
Phone: 800-738-3343
www.petedge.com

ABOUT THE AUTHOR

Shirlee Kalstone has been an internationally recognized expert on pets for over twenty years, and is the author of numerous books about dog and cat breeds, pet health care, first aid, grooming, behavior problems, and housebreaking, including *How to Housebreak Your Dog in 7 Days* (nearly 400,000 copies in print!). She is also a life-long allergy sufferer. Mrs. Kalstone has lectured on pet care and grooming across the United States, Canada, and Europe, as well as in Argentina and Japan, and she was the founder and organizer (for eighteen years) of one of the largest pet health care/grooming conferences in the world. Mrs. Kalstone and her husband have also bred and shown Poodles, Whippets, English Setters, Cocker Spaniels, Weimaraners, and Burmese and British Shorthair cats. She lives in New York City.